PSYCHOLOGY PRACTITIONER GUIDEBOOKS

EDITORS

Arnold P. Goldstein, Syracuse University
Leonard Krasner, Stanford University & SUNY at Stony Brook
Sol L. Garfield, Washington University in St. Louis

ASSESSMENT OF EATING DISORDERS

Pergamon Titles of Related Interest

Agras EATING DISORDERS: Management of Obesity, Bulimia and Anorexia Nervosa

Kirschenbaum/Johnson/Stalonas, Jr. TREATING CHILDHOOD AND ADOLESCENT OBESITY

LeBow ADULT OBESITY THERAPY

Weiss/Katzman/Wolchik TREATING BULIMIA: A Psychoeducational Approach

Related Journals
(Free sample copies available upon request)

CLINICAL PSYCHOLOGY REVIEW
ADDICTIVE BEHAVIORS

ASSESSMENT OF EATING DISORDERS

Obesity, Anorexia, and Bulimia Nervosa

DONALD A. WILLIAMSON
Louisiana State University
with C.J. Davis, Erich G. Duchmann, Sandra J. McKenzie
and Philip C. Watkins

PERGAMON PRESS
Member of Maxwell Macmillan Pergamon Publishing Corporation
New York • Oxford • Beijing • Frankfurt
São Paulo • Sydney • Tokyo • Toronto

Pergamon Press Offices:

U.S.A.	Pergamon Press, Inc., Maxwell House, Fairview Park, Elmsford, New York 10523, U.S.A.
U.K.	Pergamon Press plc, Headington Hill Hall, Oxford OX3 0BW, England
PEOPLE'S REPUBLIC OF CHINA	Pergamon Press, Room 4037, Qianmen Hotel, Beijing, People's Republic of China
FEDERAL REPUBLIC OF GERMANY	Pergamon Press GmbH, Hammerweg 6, D-6242 Kronberg, Federal Republic of Germany
BRAZIL	Pergamon Editora Ltda, Rua Eça de Queiros, 346, CEP 04011, São Paulo, Brazil
AUSTRALIA	Pergamon Press Australia Pty Ltd., P.O. Box 544, Potts Point, NSW 2011, Australia
JAPAN	Pergamon Press, 8th Floor, Matsuoka Central Building, 1-7-1 Nishishinjuku, Shinjuku-ku, Tokyo 160, Japan
CANADA	Pergamon Press Canada Ltd., Suite 271, 253 College Street, Toronto, Ontario M5T 1R5, Canada

Copyright © 1990 Pergamon Press, Inc.

Library of Congress Cataloging in Publication Data

Williamson, Donald A. (Donald Allen), 1950-
    Assessment of eating disorders : obesity, anorexia, and bulimia
nervosa / Donald A. Williamson with C.J. Davis . . . [et. al.].
      p. cm. -- (Psychology practitioner guidebooks)
    Includes bibliographical references.
    ISBN 0-08-036453-5 -- ISBN 0-08-036452-7 (pbk.)
    1. Eating disorders--Diagnosis. 2. Diagnosis, Differential.
I. Davis, C. J. (Christopher John), 1950-   . II. Title.
III. Title: Obesity, anorexia, and bulimia nervosa. IV. Series.
    [DNLM: 1. Bulimia. 2. Eating Disorders--diagnosis. 3. Eating
Disorders--therapy. 4. Obesity. WM 175 W729a]
RC552.E18W55   1990
616.85'26--dc20
DNLM/DLC   89-16193
for Library of Congress   CIP

Printed in the United States of America

The paper used in this publication meets the minimum requirements of
American National Standard for Information Sciences -- Permanence of
Paper for Printed Library Materials, ANSI Z39.48-1984

Dedication

To my parents, Miller and Mary Williamson, for all of their care, love, and support throughout the years.

Contents

Preface

Over the past ten years my staff and I have seen more than 1,000 eating disorder cases. During the same time span there has been an explosion of research related to the eating disorders. This book represents a synthesis of the knowledge (derived from both clinical experience and controlled research) that pertains to assessing the eating disorders. Most of our experience has related to the eating disorders, obesity, anorexia nervosa, and bulimia nervosa. In studying obesity we found that a substantial number of obese patients had significant problems with uncontrollable binge eating. Initially, we referred to these patients as "binge-eaters," but here have adopted a more widely used term, "compulsive overeater," to describe this population. In this volume, we have described the methodology for differentially diagnosing these four types of eating disorders and for evaluating common problems associated with each disorder. Practical, easy-to-use procedures are described which can be applied in most clinical settings. The empirical research related to each method is described in some detail, with an emphasis on documenting the experimental basis of each concept or procedure. It is our hope that the end result is a practical and useful guide for clinicians involved in the work of evaluating eating disorders. Also, students interested in quickly learning about the nature of eating disorders and procedures for assessing them should find the book quite useful.

It should be noted that this book would never have come to fruition without the assistance of my co-authors, C. J. Davis, Erich Duchmann, Sandy McKenzie, and Phil Watkins. At the time of the writing, all of these persons are advanced graduate students who have worked with me for at least four years in managing eating disorder patients. Each contributed specific chapters to the book and each has shared his or her own experiences and knowledge in writing. In many ways, they have been on the front line with these often trying cases.

The information presented here has been tried, tested, revised, and retested. We hope the reader will find that the information can be applied with a fair degree of ease so that our efforts will lead to efficient administration, planning, and decision making.

Acknowledgments

The ideas presented in this text represent the cumulative efforts of the many graduate and undergraduate students who have worked in the Eating Disorders Clinic at the LSU Psychological Services Center. The list of names is much too long to be presented here, but I would like to express true appreciation for their work conducted over the past eight years. Also, I would like to acknowledge the efforts of my wonderful secretary, Colleen Brown, for her long days and nights in preparing this text. Without her dogged determination, we would never have completed the task. Finally, the support of my wife, Stephanie, has been total and complete for all of these many years. Without that support, none of this work would have come to fruition. For the many sacrifices and times I forgot to acknowledge them, I simply say "thank you."

Chapter 1
Clinical Descriptions
of Eating Disorders

The most common types of eating disorders found in adolescents and adults are obesity, anorexia nervosa, and bulimia nervosa. During the 1980s, professionals, scientists, and the general public have shown a tremendous interest in these disorders of eating. In the United States and other Western countries, the 1970s and 1980s were associated with a strong emphasis on thinness in young women (Cash & Brown, 1987; Garner, Garfinkel, Schwartz, & Thompson, 1980). The sociocultural influence of this emphasis on thinness is generally credited as a major determinant of the apparent increased incidence of anorexia nervosa and bulimia nervosa in young women. It also partially accounts for why so many overweight adolescents and adults have been so preoccupied with losing weight. Other factors which have raised our society's consciousness about the dangers of obesity are studies which associated obesity with increased risk of medical problems, and general societal emphasis upon improved health.

As a result of two decades of research in preventive medicine, health psychology, and behavioral medicine, the public now views many health problems as preventable by changes in health habits. In particular, eating and exercise habits have been identified as behaviors which, when modified, can improve one's health status. One consequence of this change in public health consciousness is that we have begun to perceive obesity to be treatable or preventable via behavior change. As will be discussed later, this rather healthy philosophy may interact with extreme pursuit of thinness to produce anorexia and bulimia nervosa in a small subset of our population.

One result of this increased interest in eating disorders has been increased understanding of the psychological determinants of eating disorders and the development of improved assessment and treatment techniques. This book describes in detail the procedures which have been developed for assessing and diagnosing eating disorders. For information concerning the treatment of eating disorders, the reader may wish to refer to a companion practitioner's guidebook, written by Agras (1987). This first chapter will describe the clinical syndromes of obesity, anorexia nervosa, and bulimia nervosa, and will present conceptual models which can be used for developing case formulations and individualized treatment plans.

OBESITY

Simple Obesity

Obesity can be medically defined as excessive adipose (or fat) tissue (Bellack & Williamson, 1980). In clinical studies of obesity, a minimal criterion of 20% overweight has often been used. Issues related to the measurement of body fat will be discussed in more detail in Chapter 3.

Studies of the genetic contributions to obesity have shown moderate to strong hereditary influences (Price, 1987). Family studies have shown that as much as 20% to 60% of variation in body fat may be attributable to genetics. No single genetic cause has been found which can account for these influences, however.

Environmental influences upon obesity have also been found to be of significance, accounting for 20% to 30% of obesity in children and adolescents (Price, 1987). It is likely that there are genetic and environmental determinants of obesity and that both must be considered when evaluating cases of obesity.

The most commonly held theory of obesity is that it is caused by chronic positive energy balance, namely, the individual consumes more energy than is expended. Changes in weight can be understood in terms of the energy balance model shown in Figure 1.1. This simple model explains that a person gains weight when there is an excess of energy and loses weight when there is a deficit of energy. As will be discussed later in this chapter, the primary behavioral influences upon energy intake and expenditure are eating habits, activity habits, and dieting. If eating habits consistently yield excessive caloric intake or inactivity leads to a relative caloric deficit, then the individual will gradually gain weight. Research comparing the eating habits and activity levels of obese persons to those of normal weight have consistently found that obesity is maintained more by inactivity rather than by overeating (Brownell & Stunkard, 1980).

Also, it has been found that as weight increases, activity decreases (Bloom & Eidex, 1967; Chirico & Stunkard, 1960). These findings, taken

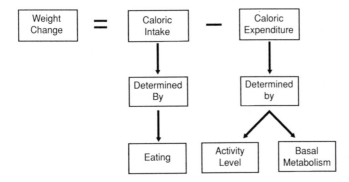

FIGURE 1.1. The energy balance model.

together, suggest that obesity may initially result from a variety of factors ranging from chronic overeating and reductions in activity to alterations in basal metabolism. However, once obesity has been initiated, alterations in activity level may help maintain obesity.

These behavioral influences upon obesity are complicated by biological mechanisms for energy regulation. There is considerable evidence that energy, and thus body weight, are regulated by homeostasis. In other words, each person has a certain set point (or body weight) which these mechanisms strive to maintain in a manner similar to how a thermostat regulates the temperature of a room (Keesey, 1980). It is generally presumed that heredity determines an individual's initial set point. This natural set point may or may not be statistically normal and may or may not be a weight level which is desired by the individual. A second influence upon the set point is nutrition. Overfeeding can lead to resetting the set point at a higher weight level. If this occurs, then weight is regulated at a higher level. In this fashion an individual may gradually gain weight and have difficulty losing weight below the new set point.

Recent research concerning the development of adipose tissue in adulthood has shed some light upon how chronic overfeeding might reset the set point at a higher level. This research (Sjostrom, 1980) has shown that overfeeding can result in the creation of new adipose tissue. Since adipose tissue (or cells) cannot be removed once created (by normal processes), the individual who is in chronic positive energy balance can only continue to gain weight and find it difficult to maintain lower weight levels. This sequence of events has been postulated to account for chronic obesity.

To fully understand how obesity develops, it is useful to conceptualize weight loss and gain in terms of caloric excesses and deficits. In terms of energy, a 1 lb. weight gain or loss is equivalent to an energy imbalance of 3500 kcal. Thus, to gain or lose 1 lb. in one week, one must have a caloric excess or deficit of 500 kcal/day. Given this formula, rapid weight gain must be caused by extreme changes in eating, such as binging or extreme inactivity from being bedridden during a chronic illness. A slow rate of weight gain is more likely caused by minor changes in eating or exercise habits. For example, drinking one "extra" nondiet soft drink (slightly over 100 kcal) every day for a year yields a total caloric excess of over 35,000 kcal/year or a gain of over 10 lbs. The following case examples illustrate how the weight histories of two cases may shed some light upon the etiology of obesity with implications for individualized treatment plans.

Case Example. Jack was a 31-year-old attorney who had graduated from law school at age 26. He had gradually gained weight from 170 lbs. at age 26 to 210 lbs. at age 31. At 5 ft. 9 in., he had been within the normal weight range for a young adult male of medium build. At 210 lbs. he was overweight and quite unhappy with his developing obesity. Each year over this five-year period he had gained 5 to 10 lbs. There had never been periods of rapid weight gain and he had no problems with weight either as a child or as an adolescent. Both of his parents were reportedly of normal weight. The history of his eating and exercise habits showed that he ate three meals per day with occasional snacks and had done so for many years. He had been an athlete in high school and had played intramural sports in college and law school. He was married at age 24 after being in law school one year. After graduating from law school, only two major changes in habits were noted. First, he no longer played organized sports, such as basketball, or individualized sports, such as golf or tennis. Furthermore, he had not developed an interest in jogging, aerobics, or other leisure activities due to the demands of his law practice and new family. He and his wife had had two children in the previous five years. The second major change was in drinking habits. While in college he drank alcohol, but mostly on the weekends, at fraternity parties. In law school he had practiced similar drinking habits. After graduation, he continued drinking on the weekends, but also began having a few cocktails on most evenings after work. He was clearly not alcoholic, but his drinking bordered on being abusive, which bothered him. From this history, two primary habits were targeted for treatment: (a) development of a regular exercise program, and (b) reduction in drinking, especially during the week.

Case Example. Jean was a 17-year-old who had been diagnosed as diabetic when she was 15 years old. She now weighed 160 lbs. and at 5 ft. 4 in. was 25% overweight. Prior to age 15 she had been slightly underweight and remembered weighing about 115 lbs. Her diabetes had an acute onset. Jean, her parents, and her doctors had found her blood glucose levels to be difficult to stabilize. When the blood glucose levels were too high, she responded by taking short-acting insulin which often resulted in hypoglycemia, that is, low blood sugar, which then required that she eat in order to raise the blood sugar level. Careful analysis of her eating habits suggested that she had developed an eating and insulin regimen requiring the consumption of 2500 to 3000 kcal/day. She was very sedentary and had recently begun to snack excessively, which required taking extra units of insulin. Together, these habits were resulting in a consistent caloric excess of 150 to 300 kcal/day, leading to a weight gain of 40 lbs. over a two-year period. Based upon this history, Jean and her endocrinologist developed a treatment plan which targeted: (a) gradual increase in exercise, and (b) elimination of excessive snacking with a parallel adjustment in her insulin regimen.

Compulsive Overeating

Recent research has suggested that 20% to 40% of obese patients have significant problems with compulsive binge eating. While compulsive binging is also found in normal weight individuals, existing research suggests that it is much more prevalent in obese populations (Marcus & Wing, 1987). In their discussion of the diagnosis of the *syndrome* bulimia nervosa, Fairburn and Garner (1986) suggested that the term bulimia be used to refer to the *symptom* of binge eating. Williamson, Kelley, Cavell, and Prather (1987) suggested that the term binge-eater be used to refer to bulimics who met the 1980 DSM-III criteria for bulimia, but had no history of purging, that is, they had problems only of compulsive binge eating. More recently, Schlundt and Johnson (in press) have proposed that this pattern of disordered eating be termed *compulsive overeater*. We have adopted this terminology, but feel that more stringent diagnostic criteria must be established if it is to be a meaningful term. Table 1.1 presents a proposal for diagnostic criteria for compulsive overeating. These criteria are a modification of the original diagnostic criteria for bulimia presented in the *Diagnostic and Statistical Manual of Mental Disorders*, 3rd ed. (DSM-III-R; American Psychiatric Association, 1980). In essence these criteria describe a syndrome of uncontrollable binge eating without extreme weight control behaviors such as purging or starving. This type of patient recognizes that the binge eating is abnormal and experiences negative affect after binging, which may precipitate further binging.

Williamson and colleagues have studied this compulsive binge-eating syndrome in a series of studies (Davis, Williamson, Goreczny, & Bennett, 1989; Prather & Williamson, 1988; Williamson, Prather, Goreczny, Davis,

Table 1.1. Proposed Diagnostic Criteria for Compulsive Overeating

---

A. Recurrent episodes of binge eating at least twice per week for 3 months (rapid consumption of a large amount of food in a discrete period of time, usually less than two hours).
B. At least three of the following:
   1. Consumption of high-caloric, easily ingested food during a binge
   2. Inconspicuous eating during a binge
   3. Repeated attempts at dieting in an effort to lose weight
   4. Negative affect often sets the occasion for binge eating
   5. Frequent weight fluctuations greater than 10 pounds due to alternating binging and dieting
C. Does not use extreme methods to lose or control weight, that is, self-induced vomiting, severely restrictive dieting, starvation, laxative or diuretic abuse, or extreme exercise habits.
D. Awareness that the eating pattern is abnormal and fear of not being able to stop eating voluntarily.
E. Depressed mood and self-deprecating thoughts following eating binges.
F. Does not evidence body image disturbances other than body size dissatisfaction.
G. The bulimic episodes are not due to anorexia nervosa, bulimia nervosa, or any known physical disorder.

Adopted from the American Psychiatric Association (1980) diagnostic criteria for bulimia.

& McKenzie, 1989). In a diagnostic study, Williamson, Prather, et al. (1989) found that compulsive overeating was a syndrome which could be reliably differentiated from simple obesity as well as bulimia nervosa.

A typical case of compulsive overeating presents with a problem of at least moderate to severe obesity. In a sample of over 50 patients, we found the average compulsive overeater to be about 60% overweight, with an average age of about 32 years at the time of presentation for treatment. A majority were women. They described problems of binging with frequencies ranging from every day to once or twice per week. Generally the binges were rather large and consisted of carbohydrates and junk foods. Typical binges were (a) a gallon of ice cream, (b) a dozen doughnuts, (c) several hamburgers, or (d) boxes or bags of cookies or chips. Most of these binges occurred in secrecy and were scheduled, such as in the afternoon after school or work. Often, family or friends believed that the individual was dieting since they typically professed to be on a diet and publicly followed the diet. Yet, they continued to gain weight at a moderate to rapid rate.

These studies have found that these compulsive overeaters seldom purge using self-induced vomiting, diuretics, or laxatives. They do, however, report using dieting and occasionally resort to using diet pills (usually nonprescription) to control their eating. Also, they do not have body image disturbances similar to bulimia and anorexia nervosa (Davis et al., 1989). Because compulsive overeaters are usually overweight, they are typically dissatisfied with body size. They do not, however, distort body size, nor do they prefer an unrealistically thin body size. These characteristics clearly distinguish the compulsive overeater from bulimia nervosa.

Studies of secondary psychopathology (Marcus & Wing, 1987; Prather & Williamson, 1988) have found compulsive overeaters to have secondary problems similar to that of bulimia nervosa. In particular, a majority of these patients are depressed and are often diagnosed as dysthymic. Personality disorders such as dependent, avoidant, and passive-aggressive are also often diagnosed. Thus, these cases generally have problems of eating as well as other clinical problems which interact to produce chronic obesity and unhappiness. The following case example illustrates the complexity of compulsive overeating in contrast to simple cases of obesity.

Case Example. Gwen was a 33-year-old mother of three children. She had been divorced for five years. She weighed 240 lbs. at a height of 5 ft. 5 in. Her history indicated no problems with her weight until after her first pregnancy at age 21. She had married when she was 19 years old. Marital problems developed over the first several years and intensified after the birth of her first child. Her husband drank abusively and often left her at home alone. During periods of loneliness, boredom, and depressed mood, she found that eating comforted her emotional state. This excessive eating resulted in gradual weight gain from about 120 lbs. at age 20 to about 160 lbs. by age 25. During this period, all three children were born.

During her early 20s, Gwen went on several crash diets involving very restrictive eating. She would become very hungry after several days of eating only one small meal per day and would inevitably break the dieting by eating snacks, especially sweets or cereals. After violating her dietary rules, she would usually think, "well, I might as well just go ahead and eat." This sequence of events inevitably led to binges which were done in complete secrecy. Typical binges included eating several boxes of cookies or cereal, ice cream, and/or candy. She was careful to hide the boxes or wrappers so that her husband could not see them.

Gradually, over the next eight years, she became more obsessed with binging. She began to hoard food and plan daily binges. Her marital problems and depression continued to worsen. Her depression was treated using antidepressant medication and she and her husband entered marital therapy, which lasted until the therapist recommended that he be treated for alcoholism. He refused this recommendation and the marriage ended 18 months later.

After the marital separation, Gwen found employment as a sales clerk in a convenience store. Her binging began to take on a more ritualistic form. Each day she ate nothing for breakfast or lunch, but would purchase candy bars, ice cream, and other snack foods, which she would eat in her car as she drove home. The binge foods were eaten very quickly and she disposed of all wrappers, containers, and so forth before arriving home. She felt very guilty about this binging since it had led to extreme obesity by the age of 33 years.

She had become chronically depressed over the years and was diagnosed as dysthymic. She had a very limited social life. She never dated and since her family lived in another area, she seldom visited them. She had a few friends, but most of her time was devoted to working and caring for her children. When she was especially upset or depressed, this set the occasion for binging at home. Recently, she had begun to awaken during the night and found that she could return to sleep only afer eating.

Gwen is a classic example of compulsive binge eating. She was referred to a comprehensive program for compulsive overeating and depression. Treatment of such cases must be broad-based, focusing on eating habits as well as other psychological problems.

ANOREXIA NERVOSA

The syndrome of anorexia nervosa has been recognized in the medical literature as a psychiatric syndrome for more than 100 years (e.g., Gull, 1874). The primary clinical feature of anorexia nervosa is extreme weight loss which can be life-threatening. This weight loss is due to extremely restrictive eating and, in most cases, excessive exercise and/or purgative behavior, such as self-induced vomiting or laxative abuse. This behavior is driven by an extreme fear of weight gain and a strong preference for thinness. Also, most anorexics display distortion of body size, which worsens as weight increases, resulting in further restrictive eating. This distortion of body size manifests itself as a perception of being fat despite being thin. Anorexics are generally very sensitive to minor fluctuations in weight or body size, such as noticing slight changes in the tightness of clothes. Some of the physical consequences of severe weight loss and restrictive eating are (a) cessation of the menstrual cycle (amenorrhea), (b) loss of hair, (c) lowered body temperature, and (d) dry skin, due to dehydration.

Extreme behavioral habits to lose weight and to prevent weight gain, such as starvation or purging, are caused by the anorexic's fear of weight gain and body image disturbances (Schlundt & Johnson, in press). The fear of weight gain can be conceptualized as a type of obsession with thinness. Each time the anorexic loses more weight, this obsession intensifies, driving even more extreme weight control methods. For these reasons, most authorities agree that the treatment of anorexia nervosa must emphasize modification of fear of weight gain in addition to changing eating habits and gaining weight.

The current revision of the *Diagnostic and Statistical Manual of Mental Disorders* (DSM-III-R; American Psychiatric Association, 1987) defines anorexia nervosa using the following criteria:

1. Refusal to maintain body weight above 15% below that which is expected
2. Extreme fear of weight gain despite being significantly underweight
3. Disturbance in body image, for example, feeling fat even though the individual is underweight
4. In females, amenorrhea for at least three consecutive menstrual cycles

These diagnostic criteria reflect research on the psychopathology of anorexia nervosa which suggests that fear of obesity and body image disturbances play a major role in the etiology and maintenance of this eating disorder. Some (e.g., Schlundt & Johnson, in press) have objected to inclusion of amenorrhea as one of the essential characteristics of anorexia nervosa since it is generally thought to be directly caused by weight loss. The following case example illustrates typical characteristics associated with anorexia nervosa.

Case Example. Lynn was an 18-year-old high school senior. She was an excellent student, usually making all As. Her parents were affluent; her father was a lawyer and her mother a homemaker who was active in civic organizations. She had two older siblings, a brother (age 24 years) and a sister (age 22 years). Both had been good students and were high achievers.

Lynn had been a popular child throughout childhood, but was somewhat shy. Also, she had always been a little overweight, something which her parents had often criticized. Her problems related to anorexia could be traced back to about age 14. At this time, she was approximately 15 lbs. overweight at about 130 lbs. She began dieting with some of her friends and took up jogging as a form of exercise. Her parents reinforced these efforts by praising her and promising the purchase of new clothes once she had lost weight. She was able to lose 15 lbs. in about two months by eating only once per day and jogging from 2 to 5 miles per day. She was very pleased with herself and received many compliments from friends, family, and teachers.

Once she tried to begin eating normally, she immediately gained a few lbs., which was very distressing. She again resumed restrictive eating habits and was able to maintain a weight between 115 and 120 lbs until age 16 years. Her eating habits became more and more rigid over time. She tried to eat no more than two meals per day, but found that she was obsessed with eating and binged frequently. This binging frightened her very much and she usually responded by exercising vigorously. Also, she occasionally used laxatives after binging, taking two or three at a time. By the time she was 17, she had found that it was easier to control her weight by simply not eating. By starving herself, she no longer felt hungry and did not have to fear binging and weight gain. She rapidly lost weight using these methods and her parents were alarmed. She remembers that once her weight was below 110 lbs., she thought, "I'll never weigh over 110 lbs. ever again." She did not, however, wish to lose further weight. When she tried to eat three meals per day, as her parents insisted, she immediately gained to 111 lbs. She reacted by increasing her exercise and skipping meals. Her parents began applying pressue to eat and it was at this time that she discovered self-induced vomiting after reading an article about bulimia nervosa. Now she could eat to please her parents, but could secretively purge in order to lessen her fears of weight gain. She lost weight to below 105 lbs. and her parents contacted the family doctor. He could find no medical cause of Lynn's weight loss and suggested that she see a psychiatrist because anorexia nervosa was suspected. The psychiatrist confirmed that Lynn was developing anorexia nervosa and prescribed an antidepressant and began weekly psychotherapy sessions.

Over the next year, Lynn became more openly resistant to eating and gaining weight. She became defiant when her parents demanded that she eat and constantly attempted to deceive them by skipping meals, eating very small portions, sliding her food around her plate and hiding it without eating. Purgative behavior continued on a daily basis. Her grades began to decline. She became socially isolated and depressed. Also, family relations suffered; meals became a time of tension and frustration. After a year of unsuccessful outpatient treatment, Lynn was referred to an inpatient treatment program for eating disorders. Her weight at admission to the hospital was 98 lbs. She had not menstruated for six months and was in poor health. She and her parents were informed that she would likely require a minimum of eight weeks of inpatient treatment followed by several years of intensive outpatient therapy for eating disorder problems.

BULIMIA NERVOSA

The syndrome of bulimia nervosa was not identified until the 1960s and 1970s. Prior to this period, the"binge-purge syndrome" was considered to be an atypical form of anorexia nervosa. During the 1960s and 1970s, the syndrome was variously called dietary chaos syndrome, bulimarexia, and dysorexia (Schlundt & Johnson, in press). In 1980, the

American Psychiatric Association adopted the term bulimia. The diagnostic criteria for bulimia emphasized binge eating and negative affect after binging. As noted by Williamson et al. (1987), this definition did not require purgative behavior for a diagnosis of bulimia. Russell (1979) presented an alternate set of diagnostic criteria for a syndrome he termed bulimia nervosa. This syndrome had three primary characteristics: (1) strong urges to binge, (2) use of purgative methods to avoid weight gain, and (3) fear of weight gain.

During the 1980s, a debate waged over the best diagnostic criteria for this "binge-purge syndrome" (Fairburn & Garner, 1986). In 1987, the American Psychiatric Association adopted a modification of the Russell criteria and adopted the name bulimia nervosa. These criteria require the following characteristics:

1. Repeated episodes of binge eating.
2. Lack of control over eating during binges.
3. Frequent use of purgative behaviors, self-induced vomiting, laxative or diuretic abuse, restrictive dieting or fasting, or excessive exercise, to prevent weight gain.
4. Binging must occur at a frequency of at least twice per week for a minimum of three months.
5. Overconcern with body shape and weight which is very persistent.

These diagnostic criteria do not directly specify fear of weight gain. They do, however, note that fear of weight gain motivates purgative behavior, which implies that fear of weight gain is a characteristic of bulimia nervosa. Others (e.g., Fairburn & Garner, 1986; Schlundt & Johnson, in press) have suggested anorexia and bulimia nervosa are best conceptualized as two syndromes with one underlying dysfunction, which has been termed intense fear of "fatness" and overconcern with body size. Williamson, Davis, Goreczny, and Blouin (1989) have also shown that bulimia nervosa is associated with disturbances of body image. Bulimia nervosa was found to be characterized by body image distortion and extreme preference for thinness, which produces increasing dissatisfaction with body size as weight increases. Similar findings have also been reported for anorexia nervosa (see Chapter 4). These findings suggest that fear of "fatness" and disturbances of body image may be the principal commonalities of anorexia and bulimia nervosa. In summary, research evidence is accumulating which suggests that anorexia and bulimia nervosa may be a unitary disorder with fear of weight gain and/or body image disturbances as the primary underlying condition(s). This conclusion is hardly surprising since it is well established that many bulimics have had previous episodes of anorexia and many anorexics develop bulimia.

There is considerable variability in the behavioral characteristics of bulimia nervosa. In particular, the characteristics of binging vary considerably. The "classic" binge is typified in the DSM-III-R description, namely, rapid consumption of a large amount of food in a discrete period of time. However, all binges do not involve eating large amounts of food. Instead, the bulimic must feel that she or he has "overeaten" (Schlundt & Johnson, in press). For example, in some cases eating small amounts of "forbidden foods" will be treated as a binge and will cause a negative emotional reaction which often precipitates purging (Ruggiero, Williamson, Davis, Schlundt, & Carey, 1988). In some cases, binging may occur predominantly at night, after falling asleep. This night binging (Williamson, Lawson, Bennett, & Hinz, 1989) usually occurs after the person is awakened from sleep and experiences a very strong urge to binge. A belief that sleep cannot be resumed unless binging occurs usually develops so that the person feels compelled to binge in order to reduce the urgent feelings and to fall asleep again. Night binges have sometimes been described as occurring while in a dreamlike state where the person is only vaguely aware of his or her actions. Eating during these binges is often quite bizarre, such as eating frozen fish sticks or a loaf of bread. In studying several cases of night binging we have found no physical or biological basis for the pattern of behavior. In all cases, an obsessive-compulsive pattern of awakening, feelings of urgency to binge, and binging to relieve these feelings and return to sleep was found.

Also, there is considerable variation in purgative behavior. The most common form of purging is self-induced vomiting. This habit requires using a finger or some object to stimulate the vomiting reflex. In some cases, vomiting may become more voluntary in that simply flexing of abdominal muscles can induce vomiting. In rare cases, the bulimic may lose control over vomiting and may begin to reflexively vomit all food that is eaten. It should be noted that the bulimic usually does not experience feelings of nausea prior to vomiting, which is an important diagnostic sign for differentiating psychogenic vomiting from bulimia nervosa. The second most common form of purgative behavior is abuse of laxatives. In most cases, laxatives are taken immediately before or immediately after binging. Usually, 2 to 5 laxatives are taken at a time. Some cases, however, take large amounts of laxatives. We have seen many cases that take more than 15 at one time and a few cases who occasionally take as many as 50. As noted by Williamson, Davis, and Ruggiero (1987), laxative abuse can result in severe dehydration and depletion of electrolytes, especially potassium (known as hypokalemia). Other forms of purging are diuretic abuse, vigorous exercise, and strict dieting or fasting. Bulimics also commonly use medications to control their hunger/appetite. One of the most dangerous purgative methods is inducement of vomiting by taking emetics such as syrup of ipecac. A variation of self-induced vomiting is rumination (Williamson, Lawson, et al., 1989). Rumination has been found to be associated with bulimia nervosa. Instead of vomiting the ruminator will regurgitate food that has been swallowed into the mouth. This regurgitated food is chewed and then reswallowed. This pattern may persist for a few seconds to a few minutes. Related to this habit is the behavior of chewing food, but spitting it out before swallowing it.

Case Example. Sharon was a 21-year-old college student. She was an attractive young woman at 5 ft. 4 in. and 123 lbs. She presented for treatment with problems of frequent binging and purging. She lived alone in an apartment near campus. Each day she skipped breakfast and seldom ate lunch. By the time she arrived home from school, she was very hungry and she usually binged on snack foods such as cookies, ice cream, soft drinks, and milk. She typically ate large quantities of these foods, such as a gallon of ice cream and a bag of cookies. She immediately purged after these binges, usually within 15 minutes of completing the binge. She reported that she would never binge unless she could purge and always binged while alone. After purging she felt "relieved." Within a few hours, the craving for food began again. She would then purchase fast foods, such as hamburgers, french fries, or fried chicken, and eat large quantities of these foods. She would again purge these foods. After studying for awhile, Sharon would often binge on sweets such as doughnuts, cereal, or bread. Again, she would immediately purge these foods. Once she began to binge she felt that she had no control over her eating, which is why she tried to skip breakfast and lunch. When questioned about fear of weight gain, she reported that she would "die rather gain even a few pounds." She also noted that she was unhappy with her current weight level and wanted to lose at least 10 lbs. In particular, she was unhappy with the size of her thighs and waist, claiming her stomach "protruded too much," especially after eating. When asked whether she would eat even small amounts of "fattening" foods without purging, she emphatically stated that she would not.

Her history showed that she had never been obese as a child or as an adolescent, but had gained a few pounds after entering college at age 18. She responded to this weight gain by dieting and losing 5 lbs. This pattern of modest weight gain and weight loss persisted for about one year. During this period she began to occasionally binge. After feeling that she was losing control over her eating, she attempted to induce vomiting after binging. At first, this was very difficult, but she was eventually able to do it more easily. Gradually, over the next two years, her binging and purging increased in frequency until the pattern described earlier became stable.

During this three-year period, Sharon became more depressed and felt that she was losing control of her life. She became more socially isolated and dated less frequently, in part because dating often involved eating without the opportunity to purge. Her parents, who lived in another city, were unaware of her eating disorder. She described her relationship with them as satisfactory.

Sharon is a classic example of bulimia nervosa. Her binges were frequent and involved eating large amounts of food. She purged after binging and was preoccupied with body size and weight. Our experience with cases such as this is that while they may be successfully treated as an outpatient, inpatient treatment is often required to assist them in gaining control over binging and purging.

CONCEPTUAL MODELS

A diversity of conceptual models have been developed for the eating disorders. These formulations have ranged from psychoanalytic (Bruch, 1973) to biological (Pope & Hudson, 1985). A review of these many theoretical models is beyond the scope of this book. Instead, descriptive conceptual models will be presented for obesity, compulsive overeating, anorexia nervosa, and bulimia nervosa. These conceptualizations are designed to aid the process of assessment and case formulation, which leads directly to the development of individualized treatment plans. In order to conceptualize eating disorders, one must understand both etiological and maintenance factors, that is, events which lead to the development of a specific eating disorder and variables which maintain the disorder once it has developed. The following sections present models which reflect current research knowledge about the psychopathology of these eating disorders.

An Etiological Model for Eating Disorders

The etiological model shown in Figure 1.2 is based upon a preponderance of research which has shown that obesity or "fatness" is a primary antecedent condition of the eating disorders. What causes obesity is still widely debated. As noted earlier, the genetic influences of obesity are well established. They do not, however, account entirely for the development of adiposity. For many years, it was widely believed that a person's total fat tissue or adiposity was established rather early in life and that early nutritional influences, in addition to genetics, were the primary determinants of obesity. Recent research (Sjostrom, 1980) has shown that later nutritional influences can result in the "fattening" of existing adipose tissue and the development of new adipose cells. These findings account for

SOCIOCULTURAL EMPHASIS UPON THINNESS

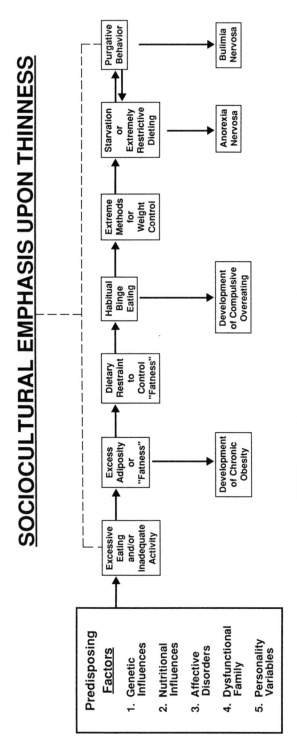

FIGURE 1.2. Etiological model for eating disorders.

the development of excessive weight in adults who were of normal weight at younger ages. Affective disorders clearly can affect appetite and activity level by either increasing or decreasing it (American Psychiatric Association, 1987). In cases where appetite is increased and/or activity is decreased, positive energy balance may result via increased caloric intake and/or reduced caloric expenditure. A history of affective disorders has especially been associated with the development of bulimia nervosa (Hinz & Williamson, 1987). Dysfunctional family environments during childhood and adolescence have also been implicated in the development of anorexia nervosa (Minuchin, Rosman, & Baker, 1978) and bulimia nervosa (Strober & Humphrey, 1987). Finally, there is substantial research suggesting that clinical cases of obesity, compulsive overeating, bulimia nervosa, and anorexia nervosa are associated with neurotic personality characteristics (Prather & Williamson, 1988; Schlundt & Johnson, in press; Williamson, Kelley, Davis, Ruggiero, & Blouin, 1985; Williamson, Prather, Upton, Davis, Ruggiero, & Van Buren, 1987). It is possible that these personality characteristics were a preexisting condition, though empirical evidence in support of this supposition is currently lacking.

The net result of these predisposing factors is an excess of eating (or caloric intake) relative to activity (or caloric expenditure). This is not to argue that obese persons overeat. Rather, the model proposes that for *that individual* a positive energy balance results from consuming more energy than is expended. The long-term effect of this positive energy balance is the development of excess adiposity or "fatness." The term "fatness," in this context, refers to feeling fat, which in some cases is due to obesity and in others may reflect overconcern with modest gains in weight, which are below typical criteria for obesity. In many cases, one or more family members (usually a parent) may be overweight and small weight fluctuations observed in adolescence may be interpreted as early signs of obesity. In such cases, the adolescent may never actually be overweight, but behaves as if she or he is.

In most cases, excess adiposity results in chronic obesity. Some may remain modestly overweight, while others may continue to steadily gain weight, resulting in extreme obesity during adulthood. The natural response of most overweight persons is to diet, which has the effect of suppressing basal metabolism (Perkins, McKenzie, & Stoney, 1987) and increasing the probability of further weight gain.

As depicted in Figure 1.2, when this weight gain occurs in a sociocultural climate which emphasizes thinness, especially in women, many young women will develop rigid rules of dietary restraint (Duchmann, Williamson, & Stricker, 1989). When dietary restraint is broken, which is probable given that dieting produces hunger and preoccupation with eating, the person is likely to overeat or binge. If this dietary restraint becomes habitual, then binging is also likely to become habitual. Each binge reinforces the idea that additional rigidity of dietary restraint is required to prevent weight gain. A recent study of Schotte and Stunkard (1987) found that approximately 10 percent of college age women have significant problems with binging. It is probable that many of these women go on to develop the compulsive overeater syndrome. Others develop more extreme methods for weight control. The data of Schotte and Stunkard (1987) suggest that approximately one-third of the bingers develop these more extreme methods of weight control. Fairburn and Cooper (1982) reported that these more extreme weight control behaviors tend to develop about 12 months after the initiation of habitual binging. Cases where starvation or extremely restrictive dieting is the predominant method adopted for controlling weight go on to develop the classic syndrome of anorexia nervosa. Starvation is difficult to maintain according to many bulimics, and they develop purgative habits, instead, as a method for controlling weight. Once purging is established as a habit, the classic binge-purge cycle of bulimia nervosa usually develops. The potential weight gain of binging can be prevented by purging, which further disinhibits binging. For many cases, binging and purging is alternated with starvation and dieting. Alternating periods of binging and purging or starving may last a few hours to weeks. Often the bulimic may feel that he or she is controlling bulimia by preventing binging, that is, by starving or dieting, and will often proudly report this "control" to their therapist. When starvation and binging/purging are extreme, the bulimic anorexic pattern results (Schlundt & Johnson, in press). It is for these reasons that bidirectional arrows are drawn between anorexia and bulimia nervosa and their associated weight control methods. These bidirectional arrows depict that bulimics and anorexics often shift in their behavior patterns from time to time and that the diagnosis that they receive may be in part due to the primary weight control methods in use at the time of assessment.

As a word of caution, the reader should realize that all eating disorder cases do not precisely fit this etiological model. For example, some anorexics do not report gaining weight or being overweight prior to the development of anorexia. These cases are a clear minority, however. Also, some anorexics never report a period of habitual binging. The intent of presenting this model is to describe the history of the typical case and to illustrate how these four eating disorders are related. From this perspective, all are developed from excess "fatness." Compulsive overeating emerges from the development of rigid dietary restraint. If intense fear of weight gain emerges, then anorexia or bulimia nervosa is likely to develop. This etiological model can be used as a guide for interviewing the eating disorder patient concerning the history of the problem. Also, when developing a case formulation, one should compare the patient's history to this typical etiology so that deviations from the "norm" are noted and integrated into the formulation.

Obesity

In previous sections, the energy balance model of obesity was presented. From a psychological perspective, the simple energy balance model is an inadequate explanation for understanding obesity. In particular, it does not explain the motivational factors which determine why an individual consistently consumes more energy than is expended. The energy balance model can easily be translated into behavior since most energy consumption is determined by eating habits and much of energy expenditure is determined by activity/exercise habits. The other primary determinant of energy expenditure is basal metabolic rate (BMR). While BMR is relatively stable over time, it has been shown that it is lowered by dieting. Since dieting is a behavioral phenomenon, BMR may also be altered by psychological processes.

Figure 1.3 summarizes the motivational processes which function to increase eating and decrease activity/exercise which result in weight gain and in turn, often leads to dieting. This model is based on a basic principle of learning that short-term consequences have a stronger influence upon behavior than long-term consequences. Appetitive behaviors such as eating or drinking are prime targets for the development of compulsive habits.

Appetitive behaviors generally have immediate positive consequences such as producing good taste and immediate removal of aversive states such as hunger. These contingencies between behavior and consequences can be conceptualized as positive and negative reinforcement, which function to strengthen eating habits. The strengthening of eating habits is likely to be observed as: (a) an overall increase in the frequency and amounts of foods eaten, (b) development of strong associations between conditions which consistently precede eating (such as environmental circumstances and time of day), and (c) the development of internal stimuli which are perceived as craving or hunger which precede eating and are reduced once eating occurs. These cravings or urges to eat are assumed to be determined by classical conditioning processes which strengthen the association between antecedent conditions (conditioned stimuli) and pre-digestive responses, such as salivation, insulin secretion, and stomach motility. These conditioned stimuli are often a complex array of environment and internal stimuli. For example, urges to eat may be strongest at a particular time of day, when feeling hungry, or fatigued or depressed. The long-term consequences of overeating may be aversive or negative,

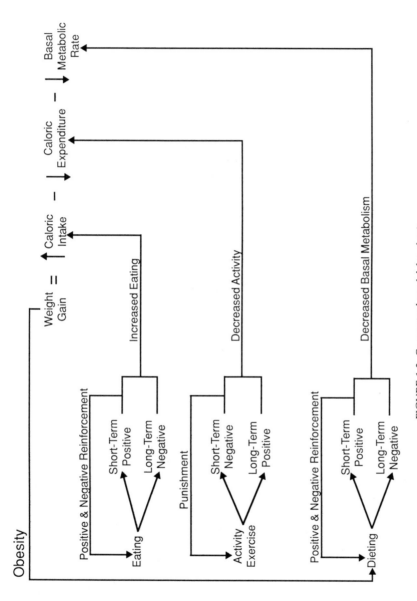

FIGURE 1.3. Conceptual model for obesity.

19

in that overeating may produce weight gain which is associated with poor health and social stigmatization. Unfortunately, the aversive consequences usually occur many years after excessive eating habits are developed and therefore have only slight influences upon eating behavior. The result of these learning processes is to increase eating and, thereby, caloric intake.

Activity level, and especially exercise, have exactly the opposite naturally occurring reinforcement contingencies. As shown in Figure 1.3, the short-term consequences of increased activity or exercise are often aversive, such as sore muscles, and are inconvenient and time-consuming. From the perspective of learning theory, this contingency between behavior and consequences can be conceptualized as punishment. Punishment has the effect of weakening or suppressing behavioral habits. The long-term consequences of exercise may be quite positive, for example, improved health, reduced weight, and greater strength. Unfortunately, these long-term consequences occur only after levels of activity or exercise are increased for a substantial period of time. The effect of these reinforcement contingencies is to produce decreased activity and, thereby, decreased caloric expenditure. Furthermore, it is assumed that environmental conditions associated with increased activity, such as an aerobics class, would be associated with negative emotions and would therefore be avoided.

If eating is increased and activity/exercise is decreased, over a period of time, the energy balance model predicts that weight gain should result. The natural response to weight gain, in today's society, is dieting. From a psychological perspective, dieting is a complex set of behavioral habits and skills. The natural short-term consequence of dieting is immediate weight loss of a few pounds, which has both positive and negative reinforcement effects. Dieting is thus strengthened as a habit. Unfortunately the long-term consequences of dieting appear to be reduced basal metabolism (Perkins et al., 1987). The most probable reason for this reduction in basal metabolism is that it is an adaptive response to starvation which has evolved over the course of mammalian evolution. In other words, homeostatic mechanisms function to conserve stored body energy when the consumption of external supplies of energy (i.e., food) is consistently low. It is presumed that this characteristic evolved as adaptive during periods of crisis such as droughts and famine. Thus, as shown in Figure 1.3, the long-term consequence of dieting is decreased basal metabolism and reduced energy expenditure, which promotes further weight gain and more difficulty in losing weight.

Figure 1.3 summarizes these behavioral determinants of obesity. This model assumes that as these three habits are strengthened, positive energy balance increases, leading to chronic obesity. The conceptual model in no way dismisses the influence of genetic or biological determinants of obesity. Instead, it is offered as a conceptual guide for understanding the psychological/behavioral causes of obesity.

Compulsive Overeating

Using the definition of compulsive overeating described earlier, we have found that a majority (about 70%) of compulsive overeaters are obese, that is, 20% or more above normal weight. It is assumed that the conceptual model of weight regulation shown in Figure 1.3 also applies to obese compulsive overeaters. What differentiates compulsive overeaters from more traditional cases of obesity is that the compulsive overeater has significant problems with uncontrollable binge eating. A study by Telch, Agras, and Rossiter (1988) found that binge eating increases as a function of increasing adiposity. This finding suggests that some portion of the obese population has significant problems with compulsive binging and that the problems of these compulsive overeaters may be different from a simple energy imbalance and resulting obesity.

The conceptual model of Figure 1.4 describes the likely determinants of compulsive overeating. This model is derived from recent research from our laboratory as well as others. The model postulates that the core psychopathology of compulsive overeating is enclosed with the dashed lines forming an elipse. Secondary problems are depicted as outside the core psychopathology and are assumed to exacerbate problems with binge eating, and they are assumed to worsen as a function of increasing problems with compulsive overeating. The bidirectional arrows are used to depict this reciprocal interaction between primary and secondary psychopathology.

Dietary restraint theory is postulated to play a major role in the maintenance of compulsive overeating. It should be recalled that the etiological model shown in Figure 1.2 postulated that binge eating is most likely to emerge after the development of dietary restraint rules to control obesity. The conceptual model of Figure 1.4 elaborates on this proposition to explain how compulsive binge eating is maintained. Dietary restraint is postulated to result in biological energy deprivation, hunger, and craving for food. Most persons will break their restraint under these conditions, which leads to binging in those characterized by high dietary restraint (Polivy & Herman, 1985). This effect was recently demonstrated in a laboratory study conducted by Duchmann et al. (1989). Although not shown in Figure 1.4, it is assumed that this binging is positive and negatively reinforced in the manner described in the conceptual model related to obesity (Figure 1.3). An additional consequence of binging is guilt about overeating and concern about weight gain. The response of the compul-

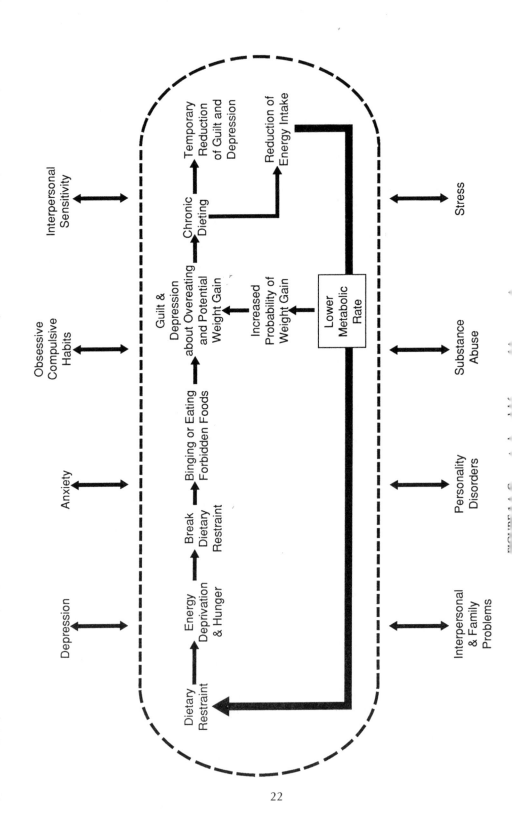

22

sive overeater to these emotional consequences is introduction of dieting, which reduces guilt, but also reintroduces dietary restraint and lowers basal metabolic rate, as discussed in the previous section. The byproduct of lowered metabolism is increased probability of weight gain, which exacerbates concerns regarding the further development of obesity. Thus, the core psychopathological model proposes that once the compulsive overeater develops rigid dietary restraint rules, a vicious cycle of psychological and biological events serve to strengthen compulsive binge eating and worsen obesity.

Secondary psychopathology, as noted earlier, is assumed to interact with core psychopathology. This interaction is postulated to be bidirectional in that as a secondary problem worsens, binge eating should worsen. This interaction is assumed to be reciprocal in the manner suggested by Hinz and Williamson (1987) for bulimia and depression. The secondary problems shown in Figure 1.4 are not meant to be an exhaustive list of other problems associated with compulsive overeating. Instead, they are simply the secondary psychopathology most commonly found in empirical studies of compulsive overeating (e.g., Marcus & Wing, 1987; Prather & Williamson, 1988; Williamson, Prather, et al., 1989). More complete discussion of these secondary problems is presented in Chapter 5.

The conceptual model of compulsive overeating shown in Figure 1.4 can be used as a guide for assessment. The model suggests that the examiner should focus upon behavioral analysis of core psychopathology and evaluation of the extent to which secondary psychopathology interacts with core psychopathology.

Anorexia Nervosa

The etiological model shown in Figure 1.2 postulates that anorexia nervosa develops after an individual begins to use extreme methods for controlling weight. Some of these persons adopt starvation or extremely restrictive dieting and develop the classic syndrome of anorexia nervosa. Others adopt purgative methods and develop bulimia nervosa. About 50% of anorexics adopt both purgative and starvation as weight control methods and thus have both anorexic and bulimic characteristics.

The conceptual model for anorexia nervosa, which is illustrated in Figure 1.5, is constructed to explain the classic restrictor type of anorexia nervosa. The same conceptual scheme used for compulsive overeating is utilized here. The core psychopathology of anorexia nervosa is depicted within the elipse formed by dashed lines. Secondary psychopathology is shown outside the core syndrome and is assumed to interact with core psychopathology in a reciprocal manner. In the case of anorexia nervosa, however, a primary underlying problem is postulated to drive the core psychopathology of anorexia nervosa. In the model of Figure 1.5 the pri-

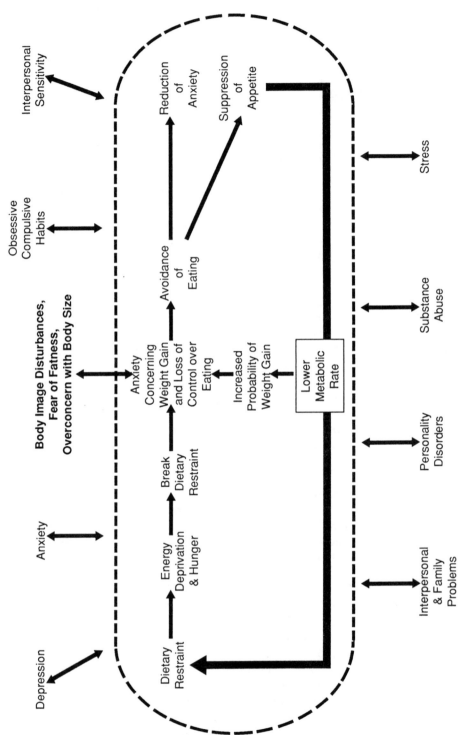

FIGURE 1.5. Conceptual model for anorexia nervosa.

mary underlying factors associated with anorexia nervosa are *body image disturbances, fear of fatness, and preoccupation with body size.* It is postulated that these characteristics are highly correlated and reflect some more central characteristic which has yet to be clearly formulated in theoretical language. A more complete discussion of the literature pertaining to this problem will be presented in Chapter 4. For the purposes of understanding the conceptual model shown in Figure 1.5, this underlying characteristic must be considered to be a type of irrational fear or obsession which increases anxiety about weight gain when dietary restraint is broken.

The etiological model of eating disorders postulates that the development of dietary restraint is a precursor to anorexia nervosa. In most cases, binge eating is a consequence of extreme dietary restraint. The conceptual model for anorexia nervosa (Figure 1.5) is an elaboration of this principle. The immediate effect of restrictive eating is biological deprivation of energy, hunger, and craving for food, as was described for compulsive overeating. Naturally occurring events lead to breaking dietary restraint or "overeating." In the etiological stage of anorexia nervosa, this breaking of dietary restraint leads to binging, which strengthens fears of weight gain. As anorexia develops, this fear becomes more intense and binging, as defined by consuming large quantities of food, is avoided. In the bulimic anorexic, binging may occur, but is "undone" by purging. In the classic restrictor anorexic, binging *and eating other foods* are avoided, which reduces anxiety concerning weight gain. In this conceptualization, anorexia is similar to a weight phobia. Another effect of starvation is suppression of appetite. This phenomenon is frequently described by anorexics as occurring after about three days of starvation. Once it has begun, the anorexic may eat small amounts of food and continue to feel as "on a high," that is, very energetic, or "in control," not fearing loss of control over binging. This suppression of appetite enhances the ability to maintain dietary restraint and avoidance of anxiety regarding weight gain. A byproduct of restrictive eating is lowered basal metabolic rate. This effect has been documented by Stordy, Marks, Kalucy, and Crisp (1977) who found that, on the average, anorexics showed lowered resting metabolism of about 24%. The long-term consequence of lowered metabolism is increased probability of weight gain, which exacerbates the existing fear of weight gain.

Secondary problems of anorexia nervosa are similar to those described for compulsive overeating. Several important distinctions should be noted, however. The family problems of anorexics are often extreme because they often use eating as a "weapon" to openly counteraggress against the family who is trying to get them to gain weight. Also, anorexics often have a more clearly defined obsessive compulsive disorder, such as cleaning or ordering rituals. Finally, substance abuse among anorexics will almost always be noncaloric, such as drugs, and will usually be designed to suppress appetite, as in using stimulants.

The proper use of this conceptual model of anorexia nervosa is to guide the assessment process. The evaluator should assess the extent to which the patient fits the model and the extent to which secondary problems interact with core psychopathology.

Bulimia Nervosa

As suggested in Figure 1.2, the binging of bulimia nervosa generally precedes extreme weight control methods such as purging (Fairburn & Cooper, 1982). Like anorexia nervosa, the core psychopathology of bulimia usually begins after a period of dieting. Figure 1.6 illustrates the conceptual model for bulimia nervosa once it has developed as a syndrome. As was noted for anorexia, underlying factors which drive the purgative behavior of bulimia nervosa are *body image disturbances, fear of fatness, and preoccupation with body size.* Williamson, Davis, Goreczny, and Blouin (1989) have shown that at all weight levels, except extremely low weight, bulimics perceive their body size to be larger than that which they consider to be ideal. In comparison to normals, bulimics perceived their current body size to be larger than normal and preferred an ideal body size that was smaller than normal. Williamson, Davis, et al. (1989) concluded that these two characteristics may interact to yield extreme dissatisfaction and preoccupation with body size, despite the fact that most bulimics are of normal weight.

The conceptual model of bulimia nervosa shown in Figure 1.6 postulates that breaking dietary restraint leads to binge eating or eating forbidden foods. This overeating activates fears of weight gain and body image disturbances to create a great deal of anxiety and worry. These emotions are often described as a feeling of being bloated or upset (Williamson, Prather, et al., 1989). The idea that these emotions are primarily due to fears of fatness are often not recognized until some time into a therapeutic program. Purgative habits serve the function of reducing this anxiety and are thus negatively reinforced. Purgative habits also eliminate energy and nutrients that were consumed. The loss of energy results in further biological deprivation and hunger, thus continuing the cycle of binging and purging. A byproduct of purging may be reduction of basal metabolic rate, which should have the effect of increasing the probability of weight gain. If normal eating results in more rapid weight gain, the fears of developing obesity should be strengthened and avoidance of eating or purgative habits should increase in frequency and severity. Preliminary evidence in support of this prediction has been recently reported by Bennett, Williamson, and Powers (1989). This study found a negative correlation between

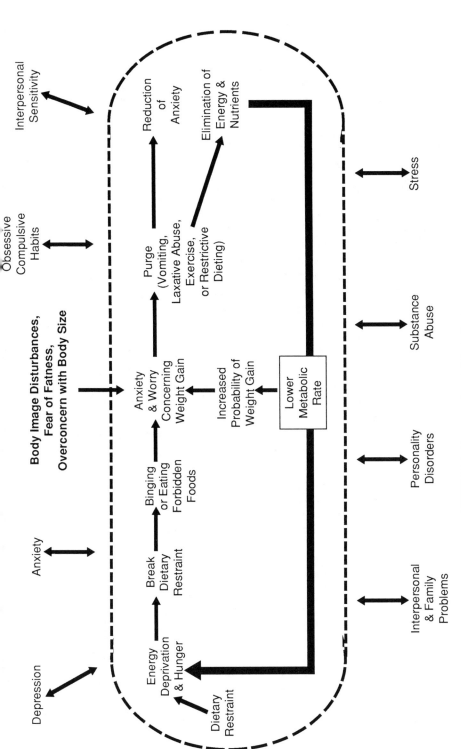

FIGURE 1.6. Conceptual model for bulimia nervosa.

27

frequency of purging and resting metabolic rate. Also, severe cases of bulimia nervosa were found to have 13% lower resting metabolism than normals. Since these data are correlational, they do not demonstrate that purging *causes* lower metabolic rate. However, the findings are suggestive that this may be the case.

A series of recent studies have presented additional evidence in support of the core psychopathology of the conceptual model shown in Figure 1.6. In support of the anxiety portion of the model, Williamson, Goreczny, Davis, Ruggiero, and McKenzie (1988) found psychophysiological evidence suggestive of anxiety following eating by bulimics. Also, Duchmann et al. (1989) and Rosen, Leitenberg, Fondacaro, Gross, and Willmuth (1985) found that when purging is prevented, bulimics avoid eating, as would be predicted by the conceptual model. Finally, Williamson, Prather, et al. (1989) reported a study which demonstrated that purging immediately reduced anxiety due to eating and that it also resulted in a dramatic decrease in serum glucose, a biological indicator of the elimination of energy and cause of increased hunger, as predicted by the model. Thus, there is considerable support for the anxiety portion of the model. In discussing compulsive overeating, research related to dietary restraint as a cause of binge eating was presented. A recent naturalistic study by Davis, Freeman, and Garner (1988) found that breaking dietary restraint was the best predictor of binging in bulimia nervosa. Williamson, Prather, et al. (1989) also found that purging resulted in overeating. These two findings suggest that perhaps binging is a function of both dietary restraint and energy deprivation as predicted by the conceptual model of Figure 1.6.

Secondary psychopathology has also been found to be associated with bulimia nervosa. In particular, depression has been fund to be correlated with severity of bulimia (Williamson, Prather, Upton, et al., 1987). Other studies have found bulimics to present frequently with significant personality problems, anxiety (Williamson et al., 1985), and interpersonal difficulties. These issues will be discussed in more detail in Chapter 5.

Summary

The conceptual models for obesity, compulsive overeating, and anorexia and bulimia nervosa were developed to assist the evaluation process. From these models, the examiner may devise case formulations and individualized treatment plans. The sections which follow discuss different aspects of the assessment process. Each section describes specific issues related to assessment and case formulation and presents specific techniques which have been found useful for diagnosing and assessing eating disorders.

Chapter 2
Differential Diagnosis of Eating Disorders

Differential diagnosis of eating disorders can sometimes be a difficult process. Cases of anorexia nervosa, bulimia nervosa, compulsive overeating, and obesity often share similar symptomatology. This chapter summarizes the assessment techniques which we have found to be most useful for diagnosing these cases. In Chapter 1, a thorough description of each diagnostic category was presented. It was noted that there are many similarities as well as differences among the four primary types of eating disorders. The similarities and differences of each diagnosis are presented in Table 2.1. Typically, anorexics are 15% or more below normal weight level, with bulimics ranging from 10% above or below normal weight. Compulsive overeaters are usually of normal weight to 20% above normal weight, and obese 20% above normal weight. Procedures for calculating percentage under or overweight are discussed in Chapter 3. With regard to binge eating, all report some incidence of binging, with bulimics and binge eaters reporting the highest frequency. Anorexics typically report episodic binging, and obese individuals binge only occasionally. To control weight, anorexics typically fast, and bulimics purge via vomiting, laxatives, diruetics, dieting, or excessive exercise. Anorexics and bulimics both report body image distortion, with compulsive overeaters and obese typically being dissatisfied only with their body size. In response to situations requiring the consumption of "forbidden" foods (foods which the individual believes are "bad," or lead to weight gain), anorexics typically avoid them, while bulimics and compulsive overeaters often binge on these "forbidden" foods. Anxiety after eating is reported by both anorexics and bulimics, but not by compulsive overeaters or cases of obesity. Negative mood preceding a binge is reported by all diagnostic groups. Finally, all groups may report additional psychopathology, with anorexics

Table 2.1. Eating Disorders: Similarities and Differences

Problem Area	OB	CO	AN	BN
Typical weight level	20% or more above normal weight	Normal weight to obese	15% or more below normal weight	Normal to 10% above or below normal weight
Binge eating	Occasional	Frequent	Episodic	Frequent
Preferred weight control method	Frequent restrictive diets	Frequent restrictive diets	Severe fasting	Purging
Body image distortion	No	No	Yes	Yes
Forbidden foods	Not applicable	Binge on them	Avoid	Binge on them, if purging is possible
Anxiety after eating	No	No	Yes	Yes
Influences of mood on binges	Yes	Yes	Yes	Yes
Presence of secondary psychopathology	Normal to Moderate	Moderate	Severe	Moderate to Severe

OB = Obese, CO = Compulsive Overeater, AN = Anorexia Nervosa, BN = Bulimia Nervosa

typically reporting the most severe pathology. Bulimia is typically associated with moderate to severe secondary psychopathology. In contrast, compulsive overeaters and obese patients typically report moderate levels of secondary problems. Use of the information in Table 2.1 may be especially helpful during the diagnostic interview. We have found that a structured diagnostic interview and a few self-report inventories specific to eating disorders are most useful for differential diagnosis. In the following sections, the use of these diagnostic procedures are discussed, and a case example is presented to illustrate how the clinician can use the data derived from these procedures to formulate an accurate diagnosis. The initial interview must be devoted to obtaining detailed information about the symptoms of eating disorders presented by a particular patient.

Several structured interviews have been developed for use with eating disorder patients. The structured interview generally has the following purposes: (a) gathering information about the patient's symptoms and goals, (b) identifying factors which maintain the presenting problems, and (c) gathering relevant historical facts. Use of a structured interview provides an efficient way to obtain specific information about the presenting problem, and insures that the essential information for making a correct diagnosis is collected. In the following section, the structured interviews which have been developed for eating disorders are described. Because none of these interview formats were designed to evaluate eating disorders ranging from anorexia to obesity, we have developed our own interview format for this purpose. This procedure is described so that the reader can apply it to clinical cases.

OVERVIEW OF STRUCTURED INTERVIEWS

A structured interview offers a systematic way to gather interview information, which can be evaluated psychometrically. Two structured interviews have been developed for assessing eating disorders. The Clinical Eating Disorder Rating Instrument (CEDRI), developed by Palmer, Christie, Cordle, Davis, and Kendrick (1987), is an instrument developed for assessing the core psychopathology of anorexia and bulimia nervosa. It was designed for the purpose of differential diagnosis of these two eating disorders. Thirty-five items, rated on a four-point scale, are used to assess behaviors, attitudes, and other symptomatology (e.g., anxiety, depression, obsessions, and psychosis) which are common to anorexia and bulimia. Interrater reliability was determined using five independent raters. For most of the items, reliability was found to be high. However, the CEDRI was developed on only 11 subjects, and no validity studies were conducted. Therefore, it is not well developed.

A second structured interview was developed by Cooper and Fairburn (1987). The Eating Disorder Examination (EDE) consists of 62 items which assess bulimic symptomatology over the last four weeks. The EDE was designed for evaluating *current* symptomatology, as opposed to assessing developmental or historical factors. Also, it was developed specifically for evaulating bulimia nervosa, and not other eating disorders. Cooper and Fairburn (1987) suggest that the EDE be utilized as a measure of treatment outcome, and do not recommend it for diagnostic purposes. Most of the items were found to have high interrater reliability.

A third structured interview, whose psychometric properties are currently being investigated, is presented here. It is called the Interview for Diagnosis of Eating Disorders (IDED). This structured interview was designed to evaluate the core psychopathology of bulimia nervosa, anorexia nervosa, compulsive overeating, and obesity, using the diagnostic criteria described in Chapter 1. The interview schedule is presented in Appendix A. The following section will present a thorough discussion of the IDED, as well as sample dialogue which may occur while using this interview format.

INTERVIEW FOR DIAGNOSIS OF
EATING DISORDERS (IDED)

The IDED is a structured interview format which was developed to systematically gather information diagnosing anorexia nervosa, bulimia nervosa, compulsive overeating, and obesity. The interview is designed for use with the patient, but many of the questions also may be used with family members in a separate interview. Discrepancies between the reports of the patient and the family should be reconciled before rating the symptoms using the scales shown in Appendix B. The interview is broken up into four major categories: *General Assessment and History, Anorexia Nervosa, Bulimia Nervosa,* and *Compulsive Overeating.* The questions are all based on the DSM-III-R criteria for anorexia and bulimia nervosa, and the diagnostic criteria for compulsive overeating discussed in Chapter 1. The diagnosis of obesity is made if the patient is 20% or more overweight for height (see Chap. 3) and by exclusion of other eating disordered symptomatology. At the end of the interview, rating scales for each of the diagnostic criteria are provided. This is discussed in Chapter 3. The rating is made by the interviewer, based on the patient's responses to questions in the interview. The following paragraphs will present a discussion of each of the sections.

General Assessment and History

The initial questions of the IDED involve gathering basic historical, medical, and family information, as well as information regarding current problems related to eating (e.g., "forbidden foods"). Questions of the IDED should be followed by additional questions tailored to the patient's answers. For example, the following dialogue may occur with a resistant patient.

Therapist: What types of problems are you currently having with eating or weight-related matters?
Patient: None.
Therapist: Why did your doctor refer you here for an evaluation?
Patient: Well, she thinks I might have an eating disorder.
Therapist: Why would Dr. Smith think that?
Patient: Because she thinks I am too skinny, and I haven't had a menstrual period in a year. The doctor talked to my parents, and they told her I never eat, but I eat. I just don't like a lot of stuff that they eat, so I don't eat with them.
Therapist: What do you typically eat?
Patient: Salads, mostly, and diet frozen dinners.

Based on this interaction, it is evident that the patient does not believe that amenorrhea, a low body weight, and restrictive eating are problematic. However, those around her are very concerned about her eating style.

Information about the patient's weight history is important, as many eating disordered patients report that they were once overweight as a child or adolescent, and that the eating disorder started during a period of dieting. Information about the course of the eating disorder is also important, so that the clinician can determine what factors have led to exacerbation and/or improvement in the person's eating disordered habits. The patient's report of medical or dental problems may lead to a referral to a physician or dentist for a complete checkup, as many patients report at least some physical problems. However, they may have been ignored by the patient until questioned about their medical state. Problems related to eating "forbidden foods" are quite common in anorexics, bulimics, and compulsive overeaters, and this information is necessary for treatment planning regarding nutritional interventions which should be made. As noted in Table 2.1, anorexics tend to avoid eating these foods and bulimics will often binge on "forbidden" foods when binging, usually followed by purging. When purging is not possible (e.g., because the bulimic is in the company of others), then avoidance of eating "forbidden" foods is the typical response of most bulimics. Compulsive overeaters tend to use these types of foods as binge foods. Typical "forbidden" foods include sweets, candy, milk products, red meats, pizza, bread, and snack foods. The evaluator may have to go through verbal listing of typical forbidden foods in order to get a complete list of what the patient will or will not eat. Also, the Forbidden Food Survey (Ruggiero, et al., 1988) can be used to establish the primary classes of foods which are feared by anorexics and bulimics. Finally, information about the patient's current family situation can be helpful for making recommendations related to the necessity of family education and/or therapy.

Anorexia Nervosa

The questions in Section II of the IDED investigate the presence or absence of anorexic symptomatology. Drive for thinness, fear of weight gain, body image distortion, and amenorrhea are assessed. In response to question 1, "Do you currently go long periods without eating?" one patient responded "Yes." However, with further questioning, this 5 ft. 4 in. 220 lb. patient noted that she often went 4 to 6 hours without eating, which to her was a long time. Another patient, 5 ft. 2 in. tall and 98 lbs., also initially responded "Yes" to the same question. However, she reported weekly fasts of 24 to 48 hours. Therefore, it is important to always follow up a yes/no response with a full description of the person's restrictive eating pattern. Information related to the history and current antecedents of restrictive eating can often help determine whether the patient is experiencing a loss of appetite due to depression versus anorexia nervosa. A more complete discussion related to the differential diagnosis of these disorders is presented in Chapter 7.

When posed with the question, "Do you feel that your weight is normal?" anorexics often report that their weight is normal, and state that they do not desire to lose any more weight. However, their responses to the next question, which asks them how they would respond to modest weight losses and gains, may show that, in actuality, they would be very pleased to lose more weight, and feel that weight gain would be treated as a catastrophe. The fourth question is designed to delineate the specific body areas which the patient may want to change (i.e., be smaller). Questions 3 and 4 are designed to evaluate diagnostic criteria related to fear of weight gain and body image disturbances. A consistent pattern of responses suggesting that weight gain produces feelings of "fatness," "bloatedness," or other negative affect, even though the patient is very thin, should be regarded as evidence in support of a diagnosis of anorexia or bulimia nervosa. Finally, the female patient may have difficulty remembering the date of her last menstrual cycle, but can often give a description of the pattern of menstrual irregularities. The DSM-III-R requires a three-month period of amenorrhea for a diagnosis of anorexia nervosa. As noted in Chapter 1, this requirement has been challenged.

Bulimia Nervosa

Section III of the IDED questions symptoms related to bulimia nervosa, with some overlap with the symptoms of compulsive overeating. Binge eating is the primary area of overlap. It is important to elicit a description of the patient's typical binge, although the patient may be embarrassed to disclose this information. Often, the patient has never described his or her binges to anyone, and so the therapist's reaction to the binge description is integral in eliciting further information from the patient. As noted in Chapter 1, many bulimics will feel that they have overeaten when they have consumed only a small portion of "forbidden" foods. Therefore, it is essential that the interview assess the patient's subjective definition of what constitutes a binge. This subjective definition can then be used to define the term *binging* for that individual. The second question relates directly to the DSM-III-R criterion related to feeling out of control during binge eating.

The third question is related to the use of extreme methods for controlling weight. Patients may deny purging, especially if they do not vomit or take laxatives. This may not be due to resistance, but to the common misperception that purging is defined only as vomiting or laxative abuse. The IDED includes questions related to diuretic abuse, appetite suppressants, dieting, and excessive exercise, so that these purgative methods are also systematically evaluated. A thorough description of the overt and covert events prior to a binge-purge cycle will provide important information for future treatment intervention. For example, a patient who binges out of "habit" (e.g., same time, same foods, without fail) will need a different intervention from the patient who binges and purges only after interpersonal conflict. The final question relates to the DSM-III-R requirement that the person has been binging at least twice per week for a diagnosis of bulimia nervosa. The requirement of "persistent overconcern with body shape and weight" (American Psychiatric Association, 1987, p. 69) should have been evaluated in the section related to anorexia nervosa.

Compulsive Overeating

Section IV of the IDED evaluates the symptoms of compulsive overeating, as defined in Table 1.1. We recommend that individuals meeting these criteria be given the DSM-III-R diagnosis of Eating Disorder Not Otherwise Specified (Eating Disorder NOS). The questions related to binge eating associated with bulimia nervosa should address the requirement of frequent binge eating. Questions 1 through 5 address the second requirement for compulsive overeating (see Table 1.1), in which the patient must meet at least 3 out of 5 criteria. Additional information is elicited about the binge eating (e.g., types of food binged on), if the patient binges alone, and emotions preceding a binge. The patient may have problems linking preceding affect to a binge. A typical interaction may go something like this.

> *Therapist:*   What emotions typically precede a binge?
> *Patient:*   I don't know, I just binge all of the time.
> *Therapist:*   Do you binge more often after a bad day?
> *Patient:*   I don't know. Well, I do binge 2 or 3 times a night after a really horrible day at work, or when the kids have been bad that day. Maybe I do binge more when I feel depressed, because I didn't binge the other day when I got a raise at work, and felt great about myself.

The remaining questions relate to feeling out of control during binges, negative affect following binges, and satisfaction with body size. Questions to rule out the presence of body image disturbances were covered in the section pertaining to anorexia nervosa.

Rating Scale for the IDED

Following administration of the IDED, a rating scale for each of the three catagories should be completed by the evaluator. This rating form is presented in Appendix B. The diagnostic criteria for anorexia, bulimia nervosa, and compulsive overeating are summarized by these ratings. The clinician rates each criterion on a seven-point scale, to determine whether the patient meets the diagnostic criteria for one or more of the eating disorders. It is usually best to make these ratings immediately after the interview, so that the patient's responses can be accurately rated. At this time, the psychometric properties of the IDED are being evaluated. Therefore, these ratings should be used as a symptom checklist in order to determine whether each of the diagnostic criteria are met. We recommend a minimal rating of 4 as a cutoff score for each diagnosis characteristic.

As noted earlier, a diagnosis of obesity should be made if the person does not meet the diagnostic criteria for anorexia nervosa, bulimia nervosa, or compulsive overeating, and is 20% or more overweight. However, many patients will not meet these diagnostic criteria, yet will have significant disturbances of eating. These patients may be diagnosed Eating Disorder Not Otherwise Specified (DSM-III-R, American Psychiatric Association, 1987), more commonly called Atypical Eating Disorder (DSM-III, American Psychiatric Association, 1980). Issues related to this diagnosis will be discussed in detail in Chapter 7.

In summary, three structured interviews for eating disorders were presented in the preceding section. The clinician must assess his or her needs to determine which is most appropriate, and meets his or her clinical needs. The structured interview, we have found, is an integral component of the assessment procedure. The IDED was developed to aid diagnosis of an eating disorder. Further interviewing may be required in order to conduct a thorough behavioral analysis and to obtain a complete history from the patient.

SELF-REPORT INVENTORIES

Several self-report inventories have been developed to assess the symptoms of eating disorders. These inventories are the Eating Attitudes Test (EAT; Garner & Garfinkel, 1979), the Bulimia Test (BULIT; Smith & Thelen, 1984), the Eating Questionnaire-Revised, (EQ-R; Williamson, Kelley, Cavell, & Prather, 1987), and the Eating Disorder Inventory (EDI; Garner & Olmstead, 1984). Each of these instruments was designed to measure some aspect of disordered eating, and a thorough discussion of each is presented below. Table 2.2 presents the mean total scores for each self-report inventory as a function of the diagnostic group. These means were computed using a large sample (n = 409) of eating disorder patients from our clinic. These data are presented so that the reader can see the pattern of test scores which is typical for these diagnostic groups. Deviations from these means can be interpreted as an index of severity.

Table 2.2. Mean Scores of Anorexics, Bulimia Nervosa, Compulsive Overeaters, and Obese Subjects on the EAT, BULIT, and EQ-R

Assessment Instruments	Purpose	X̄ Score for AN	X̄ Score for BN	X̄ Score for CO	X̄ Score for OB
EAT 24.00	Assesses anorexic symptoms	47.05	44.55	27.50	
BULIT	Assesses bulimia nervosa symptoms	89.36	125.82	111.18	86.4
EQ-R	Asseses binge eating and bulimia nervosa symptoms	42.9	52.12	46.6	39.8

AN = Anorexia Nervosa, BN = Bulimia Nervosa, CO = Compulsive Overeater, OB = Obese

Eating Attitudes Test (EAT)

Garner and Garfinkel (1979) developed a 40-item self-rating scale to assess anorexic attitudes regarding eating. The EAT is one of the most widely used assessment instruments for eating disorders. A total score of 30 or more is often used as a cutoff for anorexia nervosa. The patient is asked to rate, on a six-point scale ranging from "always" to "never," a variety of symptoms typically associated with anorexia. Reliability for the test was reported to be $r = .79$ for a clinical sample of anorexics, and $r = .94$ with a sample of anorexics and normal subjects. A positive correlation $(r = .87)$ between total EAT score and anorexic versus normal group membership was supportive of concurrent validity (Garner & Garfinkel, 1979). Gross, Rosen, Leitenberg, and Willmuth (1986) used the EAT to compare bulimia nervosa and normal controls. They found that the EAT discriminated the bulimic sample from the control sample, thus supporting the use of the EAT for assessing bulimia nervosa. Table 2.2 shows that both anorexics and bulimics score very high on the EAT. Compulsive overeaters generally have scores between that of anorexics and bulimics and that of obese patients. In summary, the EAT has been shown to discriminate bulimia nervosa from normals, and anorexia nervosa from normals, but no study has shown that it discriminates anorexia nervosa and bulimia nervosa. Thus, existing research data suggest that it is best used as a general index of anorexic characteristics, especially those concerned with fear of weight gain, drive for thinness, and restrictive eating patterns.

Bulimia Test (BULIT)

Smith and Thelen (1984) designed a 36-item test specifically designed to measure the symptoms specified by the DSM-III (American Psychiatric Association, 1980) criteria of bulimia. The BULIT requires the patient to answer questions in a multiple choice format. The questions concern binge eating, purgative behavior, negative affect, and weight fluctuations. Test-retest reliability of the BULIT was reported by Smith and Thelen (1984) to be very good (r = .87). Support for concurrent validity, using the correlation of BULIT scores with group membership (bulimia versus normals), was not as strong (r = .54). Thelen, Mann, Pruit, and Smith (1987) conducted a factor analysis of the BULIT. Six factors were derived: (1) vomiting, (2) binging, (3) negative feelings about binging, (4) menstrual problems, (5) preference for high calorie, easily ingested foods, and (6) weight fluctuations. Williamson, Prather, Davis, et al. (1987) reported that the BULIT total score was positively correlated with frequency of binging and purging, as derived from two weeks of self-monitoring. Williamson, Prather, et al. (1989) reported a study which found that the BULIT differentiated bulimia nervosa and compulsive overeaters from normals, but did not differentiate bulimia nervosa and compulsive overeaters. Table 2.2 shows that compulsive overeaters and bulimics score very high on the BULIT. Anorexics and obese subjects tend to score somewhat lower. It can be concluded that the BULIT is a valid measure of the syndrome defined by the 1980 DSM-III criteria for bulimia. Also, it is useful for ruling out anorexia nervosa. It is not very useful, however, for distinguishing bulimia nervosa from compulsive overeating.

Eating Questionnaire-Revised (EQ-R)

Williamson et al. (1987) constructed a test which, like the BULIT, was designed to measure the DSM-III (American Psychiatric Association, 1980) criteria of bulimia. It consists of 15 multiple choice items and is shown in Table 2.2. The EQ-R was originally designed as a symptom checklist, but recently has been developed as a single factor test (Williamson, Davis, Goreczny, et al., 1989). Test-retest reliability for the EQ-R has been found to be very good (r = .83). Internal consistency was also found to be quite high (coefficient alpha = .87). The EQ-R was found to be highly correlated with the BULIT (r = .80), and to discriminate bulimics from normals. A comparison of bulimia nervosa, compulsive overeaters, obese, and normal subjects found that the bulimia nervosa and compulsive overeater groups did not differ on total EQ-R scores. They scored higher than the obese group and the nonclinical sample. The obese group scored significantly higher than the normal group. Table 2.2 shows that bulimics and compulsive overeaters score highest on the EQ-R. Anorexics and obese subjects have somewhat lower scores. As noted earlier, the EQ-R was designed as a symptom checklist for bulimia. Evaluation of the reliability of each item of the EQ-R has found most items to be quite stable. Therefore, the EQ-R is best used as a check on self-report of specific bulimic symptoms. When used in this fashion, it can be a very helpful validation check for information gathered during the diagnostic interview.

Eating Disorder Inventory (EDI)

The EDI is a 64-item test constructed to measure the cognitive and behavioral characteristics of anorexia and bulimia nervosa (Garner & Olmstead, 1984). It differs from the EAT in that it is less specific to the symptoms of anorexia nervosa. The EDI requires the patient to rate his or her behavior and beliefs on a six-item scale ranging from "always" to "never." The EDI has eight scales which we have found to be positively correlated: (1) drive for thinness, (2) bulimia (e.g., binge eating), (3) body dissatisfaction, (4) ineffectiveness, (5) perfectionism, (6) interpersonal distrust, (7) interoceptive awareness, and (8) maturity fears. Using a sample of anorexics and normal subjects, internal consistency of each subscale was found to be above .80. Average item-total correlation suggested a modest degree of internal consistency among the scales (r = .63). Strong support was found for the convergent and discriminant validity of each subscale. Also, the criterion validity of the EDI subscales was investigated, using experts' ratings. Satisfactory support was found for each subscale, with correlations ranging from r = .43 to r = .68 (Garner & Olmstead, 1984).

We have found the EDI to be quite useful for evaluating the symptoms of anorexia and bulimia nervosa. In one study involving over 60 bulimics, we found mean subscale scores of bulimics to correspond very closely to the norms specified by Garner and Olmstead (1984) for anorexics. In particular, the subscales specific to eating disorder problems are quite useful for diagnostic purposes. The subscales are drive for thinness, bulimia, and body dissatisfaction. We have found the other scales, which are reportedly associated with secondary problem areas, to be less useful.

Summary

None of these self-report inventories are uniquely useful for differential diagnosis of eating disorders. All were designed for only one or two of the primary eating disorders. Both the BULIT and EQ-R were designed for diagnosis of the syndrome defined by the 1980 DSM-III description for bulimia. Neither distinguishes bulimia nervosa from compulsive overeating. Therefore, there is no one self-report inventory which can be used for diagnosis of eating disorders. Instead, a pattern of test scores in conjunction with interview data can best be used to establish an accurate diagnosis. These procedures are discussed in the next section.

INTEGRATION OF INTERVIEW
AND SELF-REPORT DATA

In using the aforementioned self-report questionnaires, we have found that a pattern of test scores emerges for each diagnostic category. Instead of relying solely on information from each total test score, the pattern of scores will lend information about the patient's symptomatology. Test scores can help interpret the index of severity of the major problem areas. For example, anorexics typically score high on the EAT, low on the BULIT and EQ-R, high on the Drive for Thinness and Body Dissatisfaction subscales of the EDI, and low on the Bulimia subscale of the EDI. This pattern indicates that there are many anorexic behaviors and cognitions (EAT), few binge eating and/or purgative behaviors (BULIT, EQ-R, and Bulimia subscale of EDI), and a high level of drive for thinness and body dissatisfaction (EDI). A cautionary note involves anorexics responding to the EQ-R. Many anorexics have found it difficult to answer the items on this test, as they refer to binge eating, which anorexics rarely engage in. Therefore, it is advisable to go over the test items immediately after the patient has taken the test, to insure that she or he has answered the test correctly.

Bulimics typically have a very simple pattern—high scores on all of these questionnaires. Compulsive overeaters score low on the EAT, high on the BULIT and EQ-R, and high on the Bulimia and Body Dissatisfaction subscales of the EDI. The Drive for Thinness subscale score is typically low. Finally, obese patients score low on the EAT, BULIT, and EQ-R, as well as the Drive for Thinness and Bulimia subscales of the EDI. Only the Body Dissatisfaction subscale is high. In the following section, four case examples are presented to demonstrate these patterns.

Case Example (Obesity). Renee was a 40-year-old female who was 5 ft. 4 in. tall and weighed 220 lbs. She was referred by her physician for treatment of her eating disorder. Renee reported that she had been obese since she was 19 years old, after the birth of her first child. Renee had been on many diets in the past 21 years, without long-lasting success. She reported eating some meals, but did not report binge eating. Her overeating was typically preceded by interpersonal conflict with her family. She reported frequent conflicts with her husband, and was very distressed about the current state of her marriage. Self-monitoring was consistent with her self-report. Renee's testing resulted in scores of 20 on the EAT, 84 on the BULIT, 40 on the EQ-R, 4 (t = 60) on the Drive for Thinness subscale of the EDI, 9 (t = 96) on the Bulimia subscale, and 15 (t = 76) on the Body Dissatisfaction subscale. Based on this information, Renee was given the diagnosis of obesity. Recommendations were made for Renee to be referred for nutritional counseling to facilitate meal planning and weight loss, as well as marital therapy for Renee and her husband.

Case Example (Compulsive Overeating). Cathy was a 28-year-old female who was self-referred for treatment of her eating disorder. Cathy was 5 ft. 6 in. tall and weighed 165 lbs. She was married and had one child. During the interview, Cathy reported frequent binge-eating epidodes, typically occurring 4 to 6 times per week. She binged in the afternoon, while her child was napping, and before her husband came home. Her binges consisted of ice cream, cookies, potato chips, and other "snack" foods. Binges occurred typically when Cathy had had a difficult time with her child, or when she had felt "cooped up" by being at home all day. The binges were very pleasurable for Cathy while she was binge eating, but she felt very badly about her "lack of self-control" after the binge. On her testing, Cathy scored a 33 on the EAT, a 112 on the BULIT, and a 47 on the EQ-R. Her EDI raw scores were a 6 (t = 69) on Drive for Thinness, 2 (t = 77) on Bulimia, and 16 (t = 79) on Body Dissatisfaction. Based on this information, Cathy was given the diagnosis of compulsive overeating, and referred for group eating disorders treatment, to focus on reduction of binging, nutritional counseling for meal planning, and weight loss.

Case Example (Bulimia Nervosa). Liz was a 19-year-old female who was referred by her parents for eating disorders treatment. She was 5 ft. 5 in. tall and 120 lbs. Liz reported that she had been overweight as a child and adolescent, and began to purge via vomiting when she was 16 years of age in order to lose weight. She began to binge, followed by purging, approximately six months later. Liz also reported taking diuretics, which she took (without her parents' knowledge) out of her father's prescription (for high blood pressure). She took diuretics approximately once per week, and vomited 2 to 3 times per day. Liz purged almost everything she ate, with the exception of very small meals, such as an apple or granola bar. Liz's scores on testing were as follows: 46 on the EAT, 129 on the BULIT, 55 on the EQ-R, 13 (90th percentile) on the Drive for Thinness subscale of the EDI, 16 (99th percentile) on the Bulimia subscale, and 19 (86th percentile) on the Body Dissatisfaction subscale. Based on this information, Liz was given the diagnosis of bulimia nervosa, and it was recommended that she enter inpatient treatment. Treatment goals were reduction of binging and purging, improved nutrition, weight maintenance, and cognitive therapy to facilitate development of rational thoughts regarding food and appropriate weight level.

Case Example (Anorexia Nervosa). Jane was a 16-year-old female referred by her physician for eating disorder treatment. Jane was in the gifted and talented program at her school and was a very good student. She was 5 ft. 8 in. tall and 115 lbs. Jane reported that she ate in a "healthy" way, but her parents and peers reported that they rarely saw Jane eat any more than a piece of fruit or a salad at any meal. She never snacked. After being presented with this information, Jane admitted that she was severely restricting her food intake, for fear of being "fat." She had been overweight as a child, but "grew out of it" at around age 12. She began her restrictive eating pattern at age 13, after noting feeling "bloated" around the time of her menstrual cycle. Her restricting became more and more severe, until present, when Jane was consuming approximately 400 calories per day. Jane's responses to self-report questionnaires yielded the following results: 50 on the EAT, 91 on the BULIT, and 40 on the EQ-R. On the EDI, Jane scored 21 (100th percentile) on the Drive for Thinness subscale, 2 (77th percentile) on the Bulimia subscale, and 20 (87th percentile) on the Body Dissatisfaction subscale. Based on this information, Jane was given the diagnosis of anorexia nervosa. It was recommended that she enter inpatient eating disorders treatment to focus on nutritional counseling for meal planning and weight gain, appropriate caloric intake, family education of eating disorders, cognitive therapy, and body image therapy.

Summary

In summary, the use of the structured clinical interview and self-report instruments can provide useful information for differential diagnosis of the eating disorder patient. However, the use of these assessment techniques can also be quite cumbersome, and overreliance on either may lead to a "can't see the forest for the trees" scenario. A certain amount of clinical judgment is required to interpret the information obtained from the interview and self-report inventories and to find the "best fit" for matching the assessment data with the diagnostic criteria for each disorder. As noted at the beginning of this chapter, anorexia nervosa, bulimia nervosa, binge eating, and obesity may share symptomatology, but with the use of the aforementioned assessment techniques, the diagnosis of an eating disorder can be made in a reliable manner. In the next two chapters, techniques for behavioral assessment and body image assessment are described. These approaches, in combination with clinical interviews and self-report inventories, are sufficient for establishing a differential diagnosis of eating disorder in most cases.

Chapter 3
Behavioral Assessment

As discussed in Chapter 2, the most common methods for assessing eating disorders are clinical interviews and self-report inventories designed to measure the cognitive, emotional, and behavioral characteristics of eating disorders. These methods of assessment have been criticized for being too removed from the specific behaviors of interest, that is, binging, purging, avoidance of eating, and so forth (Schlundt, 1989). In an attempt to obtain more direct and specific information about these behaviors and their consequences (e.g., changes in weight or body fat), a variety of behavioral assessment approaches have been developed. These approaches can be categorized as: (a) assessment of eating during test meals, (b) measurement of weight and body composition, and (c) assessment of eating and purgative habits via self-monitoring. These assessment methods are discussed in the following sections.

TEST MEAL PROCEDURES

Direct measurement of eating behavior during test meals is the quintessence of behavioral assessment of eating disorders. Earlier behavioral observation studies investigated the topography of eating in normal and obese subjects. The most frequently examined parameters included meal frequency, taste, caloric density, cognitive factors such as caloric labeling, and environmental events such as the time of day (Pudel, 1977). These studies generally failed to find differences in eating habits which distinguished normal and obese samples. They did, however, provide valuable information for developing behavioral assessment procedures which have been used in therapeutic programs for obesity. Behavior modification programs, in particular, make use of such techniques as reducing the speed of eating, drinking fluids before meals, leaving food on the plate, and limiting the number of food cues in one's environment.

More recently, investigators have used behavioral observation in studying dietary restraint in normal and obese subjects (e.g., Herman & Polivy, 1975; Ruderman & Wilson, 1979; Woody, Costanzo, Leifer, & Conger, 1981). As noted in Chapter 1, the concept of dietary restraint refers to those attitudes and behaviors adopted by an individual in order to restrict food consumption for the purpose of weight loss. It has been proposed that a variety of environmental events (e.g., emotional distress, consumption of high-caloric or "forbidden" foods) can cause an individual to "break" dietary restraint. The breaking of dietary restraint is thought to result from the violation of one or more dietary restraint rules. Such rules may dictate consumption of only a specific number of calories (e.g., 1000, 800, 500 or less), a specific number of meals (e.g., 2 or fewer meals), or specific types of foods (e.g., no sweet or high caloric foods). These rules are useful in that they give the dieter a way to structure eating behavior. However, such rules also teach dieters to adopt an all-or-none, dichotomous thinking style. Following the violation of a dietary restraint rule, dieters often feel as though they have failed in their dieting effort for the day and experience what has been referred to as the "what-the-hell" effect. Since they have blown the diet for the day, they might as well indulge themselves, and renew the diet tomorrow. Dietary restraint experiments are designed to place restrained individuals in situations where dietary restraint rules are most likely to be violated, so that the breaking of dietary restraint can be examined. For example, in a forced-consumption experiment, the subject is usually required to eat foods high in calories in order to violate the subject's restraint rules for forbidden foods and/or caloric consumption. Subjects' eating behavior in a subsequent "ad lib" eating situation is then examined for differences between restrained and normal eaters. While dietary restraint has not been able to distinguish reliably between obese and normal subjects, it has provided researchers with a possible explanation for the occurrence of frequent binge eating among dieters (i.e., restrained eaters) in that restrained eaters tend to eat greater quantities of food when dietary restraint is broken (for a review of this literature, refer to Herman & Polivy, 1980).

Although the majority of the research in this area has focused on non-clinical normal-weight and obese subjects, a recent investigation found that the role of dietary restraint may be an important factor in understanding binge eating in bulimia nervosa and compulsive overeating (Duchmann, Williamson, & Stricker, 1989). In this investigation, two clinical groups, bulimia nervosa and compulsive overeaters, were compared to a group of normal, unrestrained eaters. All subjects were first required to eat a serving of chocolate pudding, which was immediately followed by the opportunity to eat two large bowls of ice cream. Subjects were instructed to taste the ice cream in a "taste test." They could then eat as much of the ice cream as they desired. Subjects were told that the experiment required that they stay in the laboratory for 1.5 hours after eating so that bulimics would believe that purging would be impossible. The results of this investigation showed that the compulsive overeaters "binged" in the "taste test," but that bulimics did not. This finding supports the role of breaking dietary restraint upon binging, which was presented in the compulsive overeater model in Chapter 1 (Fig. 1.4). These data also suggest that binge eating in bulimia nervosa is most likely to occur when environmental circumstances allow purging.

This procedure illustrates how test meals may be employed as a behavioral avoidance test in the assessment of bulimia nervosa. As noted in Chapter 1, anorexia and bulimia nervosa can be likened to an anxiety disorder in which purging or avoidance of eating serves to relieve the anxiety that is associated with consumption of forbidden foods or large quantities of food. This fear may be evaluated by exposing the bulimic or anorexic to the feared stimulus (e.g., forbidden food) in a standardized test meal and then measuring both food consumption and self-reported anxiety. Purging must be prevented for the anorexic or bulimic to experience anxiety and, in turn, exhibit avoidance of eating. This technique can be particularly useful for assessing patients who minimize problems associated with eating in order to avoid treatment. A detailed discussion of the use of test meals to diagnose resistant patients is presented in Chapter 6.

In an attempt to establish the validity of this type of assessment procedure, Rosen, Leitenberg, Fondacaro, Gross, and Willmuth (1985) compared the eating behavior of bulimia nervosa patients to that of normal eaters in both laboratory and at-home standardized test meal situations. Bulimia nervosa subjects were informed that they should not vomit 1½ hours preceding, and 2½ hours following each test meal, and that they should eat only as much of the test meal that they could "keep" without purging. Consumption of food was measured as the percentage of calories consumed. Anxiety and urge to vomit were measured using Likert-type scales where 0 was defined as no anxiety or urge to vomit, and 100 was defined as extreme anxiety or urge to vomit. A thought sampling procedure using a tape recorder was also employed to assess thoughts associated with the laboratory test meal.

Normal subjects were found to eat significantly greater amounts (calorically) than bulimia nervosa subjects for all test meal situations. Ratings of anxiety and urges to vomit were significantly greater for bulimic subjects than for normals except in the test meal which required eating a candy bar. In this meal, bulimics ate only 12% of the candy bar verses 69% for normals. The bulimics experienced small but significantly greater urges to vomit, and no greater anxiety. In addition, Rosen et al. (1985) found that bulimia nervosa subjects who were the most anxious about eating and consumed the least food in the test meals, also had more severe problems with binge eating and vomiting at home as measured by self-monitoring of eating over a three-week period.

Targeting Forbidden Foods

In addition to learning to eat more regularly and nutritiously, it is also important for eating disorder patients to learn to eat forbidden or feared foods without binging or purging. As discussed earlier, forbidden foods are typically foods which taste good and/or are high in caloric content. Because they are associated with weight gain, they cause significant emotional problems for eating disorder patients.

In many ways, forbidden foods function as a phobic stimulus for anorexia and bulimia nervosa. Purging serves the function of "undoing" the consumption of forbidden foods in that it reduces the anxiety that is associated with overeating or eating forbidden foods. Thus, Rosen and Leitenberg (1982) have suggested that purging may actually serve to maintain binge-eating behavior in these patients and that treatment should focus on prevention of purging. In this approach, patients are exposed to (i.e., required to eat) their feared foods, but are prevented from engaging in an escape response such as subsequent purging or dietary restriction.

In the effort to reduce urges to binge and purge associated with forbidden foods, we have found it useful to have patients establish a hierarchy of foods ranging from least forbidden to most forbidden. These foods are entered onto a record sheet so that the patient and the therapist can monitor the patient's progress in learning to eat forbidden foods properly. In Figure 3.1, an example of this form is presented for a hypothetical case named Judy.

In the early stages of treatment, the patient is required to eat foods that are low on the list (i.e., least forbidden) until she or he can comfortably eat them. Progress can be assessed through the use of self-rating scales of urges to binge and purge. As treatment progresses, the patient incorporates more and more fearful foods into meals until all foods on the list can be eaten with relative comfort. For example, Figure 3.1 shows that Judy tried several forbidden foods during the first week of the treatment program. However, she still experienced significant discomfort and urges to purge after eating cereal and hot dogs. Thus, she was required to try these foods again during the second week. A check mark is not placed in the "Accomplished" column until the food can be eaten without significant discomfort. In this example, Judy has overcome her distress with many forbidden foods, but she still does not feel comfortable eating beans, peanuts/peanut butter, fried fish, cheese cake, and chocolate pudding. Dur-

NAME___Judy C.___

DATE OF INITIATION OF PROGRAM___4 - 11 - 88___

COMPLETION DATE___

		Foods	Week of Program to be eaten	Accomplished
LEAST FORBIDDEN	1.	Cereal	1, 2	✓
	2.	Turkey	2	✓
	3.	Cabbage	1	✓
	4.	Okra	1	✓
	5.	Baked Potato	3	✓
MODESTLY FORBIDDEN	6.	Hot Dog	1, 2	✓
	7.	Beans	2, 3	
	8.	Corn	3	✓
	9.	Spaghetti	3	✓
	10.	Mexican Food (Tacos)	2, 3	✓
MODERATELY FORBIDDEN	11.	Peanuts / Peanut Butter	4, 5	
	12.	Chips	3	✓
	13.	Fried Chicken	4	✓
	14.	Beef	4	✓
	15.	Fried Fish	5	
VERY FORBIDDEN	16.	French Fries	5	✓
	17.	Fried Shrimp	4	✓
	18.	Cheese Cake	5	
	19.	Pie	4, 5	✓
	20.	Chocolate Pudding	5	

___Ron Fergeson, M.A.___   ___4 - 11 - 88___
Signature of Person Completing Form   Date

FIGURE 3.1. Hierarchy of forbidden foods.

ing the ensuring weeks Judy should be required to continue to incorporate these remaining forbidden foods into her meal plan so that there will be virtually no foods that she is avoiding for fear of weight gain. Through such an exposure program, the tendency for Judy to binge and/or purge can be significantly diminished.

Assessing Treatment Efficacy

Standardized test meals can also be used to assess progress over the course of treatment. At the pretreatment stage, a meal consisting of standard servings from each of the food groups (i.e., protein, starch, fruit, vegetable) can be administered and the percentage consumed from each food group as well as overall caloric consumption can be recorded. In addition, self-rating scales can be employed to assess pre- and postmeal anxiety, and postmeal urges to binge and/or purge. Figure 3.2 illustrates a form containing sample data about test meal consumption for a bulimic patient named Ann. On this form, the patient rates her anxiety and urges to binge and/or purge. At the completion of the meal, the observer records the amounts of foods eaten which later can be used to compute caloric intake.

This figure shows that Ann ate relatively small proportions of the entree and dessert, but was able to eat significantly greater amounts of the foods that are lower in calories, which resulted in an overall low caloric consumption for the meal. Furthermore, Ann's self-rated anxiety before the meal was moderate, but rose to a very high level following eating. Urges to purge were of mild severity while urges to binge were shown to be moderate. At periodic points throughout treatment (e.g., weekly or monthly), as well as at posttreatment and follow-up, this same test meal can be administered to patients and the percentages eaten, anxiety, and urges to binge/purge can be compared to those at pretreatment in order to assess treatment efficacy and verify other assessment information. For example, following Ann's sixth week of treatment, self-monitoring data indicated that she was consuming a significantly greater amount and variety of foods at meals, but her weight had not increased. A second identical test meal was administered at this time and it was found that Ann had made virtually no progress in eating "forbidden" foods without significant anxiety and urges to purge. Information associated with the test meal is represented in Figure 3.3.

This information shows that Ann ate somewhat more of the entree and the dessert than she did during the pretreatment test meal. However, her ratings of anxiety were equivalent to those during pretreatment and her urges to purge were rated to be higher. It was clear that Ann had not experienced a decrease in her discomfort associated with the consumption of high-caloric foods. It was also determined that she was significantly overestimating the amounts and types of foods she was consuming in her self-monitoring. Thus, the rationale for learning to eat forbidden foods was reemphasized and a more focused approach was taken to expose Ann to these foods. During the final two months of treatment, Ann evidenced a gradual weight gain to a normal level and weight maintenance thereafter according to the goals of treatment. At posttreatment self-monitoring

Name: Ann S.   Date: 3-22-88

(please circle):

(Pretreatment)   Mid-treatment   Post-treatment
                        (____ months)   (____ months)

FOOD (Food Group)	AMOUNT EATEN	CALORIES
Chicken Fillet (protein)	5%	17
Bread (X2) (starch)	50%	75
Slice of Chocolate Cake (starch)	0%	0
Apple (fruit)	100%	80
Salad with Dressing (vegetable)	100%	60
TOTALS:	51%	232

Please indicate your level of anxiety prior to eating.

```
0              25            (50)           75            100
!--------------!--------------!--------------!--------------!
Not                                                      Very
At All                                                   Much
```

Please indicate your level of anxiety after eating.

```
0              25             50            75          (100)
!--------------!--------------!--------------!--------------!
Not                                                    (Very
At All                                                  Much)
```

Please indicate your urge to purge after eating.

```
0            (25)             50            75            100
!--------------!--------------!--------------!--------------!
Not                                                      Very
At All                                                   Much
```

Please indicate your urge to binge after eating.

```
0              25            (50)           75            100
!--------------!--------------!--------------!--------------!
Not                                                      Very
At All                                                   Much
```

FIGURE 3.2. Test meal data: Pretreatment.

indicated that she was eating a wide variety of foods in a nutritionally balanced fashion and there were no incidences of binging or purging. Self-report indicated a relative absence of anxiety associated with eating and greatly reduced urges to binge and purge. A test meal was administered which was identical to the two test meals previously administered

Assessment of Eating Disorders

Name: ___Ann S._____   Date: ___5-6-88___

(please circle):

Pretreatment   (Mid-treatment)   Post-treatment
                      (1.5 months)   (____ months)

FOOD (Food Group)	AMOUNT EATEN	CALORIES
Chicken Fillet (protein)	15 %	31
Bread (X2) (starch)	60 %	90
Slice of Chocolate Cake (starch)	5 %	10
Apple (fruit)	100 %	80
Salad with Dressing (vegetable)	90 %	54
TOTALS:	54 %	285

Please indicate your level of anxiety prior to eating.

```
0           (25)          50          75          100
!-------------(-!-)----------!------------!------------!
Not                                                  Very
At All                                               Much
```

Please indicate your level of anxiety after eating.

```
0            25           50          75      (    )100
!-------------!------------!------------!----(     !--!
Not                                          (    )Very
At All                                            Much
```

Please indicate your urge to purge after eating.

```
0            25         ( 50 )         75          100
!-------------!---------(-!-)----------!------------!
Not                                                Very
At All                                             Much
```

Please indicate your urge to binge after eating.

```
0            25         ( 50 )         75          100
!-------------!---------(-!--)---------!------------!
Not                                                Very
At All                                             Much
```

FIGURE 3.3. Test meal data: Midtreatment.

to Ann before and during treatment. The results of this test meal are shown in Figure 3.4.

The information in this figure indicates that Ann was able to eat significantly greater amounts of the high-caloric foods (i.e., entree and dessert) and that the associated levels of anxiety were very low. Furthermore,

Name: Ann S   Date: 7-24-88

(please circle):

Pretreatment   Mid-treatment   Post-treatment
                      (____ months)   (4 months)

FOOD (Food Group)	AMOUNT EATEN	CALORIES
Chicken Fillet (protein)	95 %	323
Bread (X2) (starch)	70 %	105
Slice of Chocolate Cake (starch)	100 %	200
Apple (fruit)	80 %	64
Salad with Dressing (vegetable)	95 %	57
TOTALS:	88 %	749

Please indicate your level of anxiety prior to eating.

```
 0            25            50            75           100
:---/-----------:-------------:--------------:------------:
Not                                                    Very
At All                                                 Much
```

Please indicate your level of anxiety after eating.

```
 0           (25)           50            75           100
:-----------:---:----------:-------------:-------------:
Not                                                   Very
At All                                                Much
```

Please indicate your urge to purge after eating.

```
 0         (   ) 25          50            75           100
:--------:---:-----------:-------------:-------------:
Not                                                  Very
At All                                               Much
```

Please indicate your urge to binge after eating.

```
 0            25            50            75           100
:--:-----------:-------------:-------------:-----------:
Not                                                  Very
At All                                               Much
```

FIGURE 3.4. Test meal data: Posttreatment.

ratings of her urges to binge and purge were greatly reduced. This information provided rather direct support for the self-monitoring and self-report data, and the decision was made to place Ann into a maintenance treatment program in which she gradually would be faded from eating disorder therapy.

MEASUREMENT OF WEIGHT AND
BODY COMPOSITION

Obese and anorexic individuals are, by definition, abnormal in weight, while bulimics may be under, over, or normal in weight. In addition, a common misconception is that the term "compulsive overeater" is synonymous with obesity. However, only about 70% of the compulsive overeaters seen in our program are found to be obese. Thus, the assessment of current and ideal body weight is particularly important in classifying eating disorder patients, and in establishing goals for nutritional therapy.

Typically, an individual's current weight is compared to his or her ideal weight, which is taken from a set of normative height and weight tables. It should be noted that there is considerable debate about the proper estimates of ideal weight for an individual and that different actuarial tables yield considerable variability in estimates of ideal weight. The most frequently referenced weight table is that compiled by the Metropolitan Life Foundation (1983). The weight ranges in this table vary according to body frame (i.e., small, medium, and large). From this table, ideal weight of the person is estimated and used to calculate the percentage of difference between current and ideal weights using this formula:

$$\% \text{ Diff. from Ideal Weight} = \frac{\text{Current Weight} - \text{Ideal Weight}}{\text{Ideal Weight}} \times 100$$

As an example, a female of medium build who is 5 ft. 3 in. tall has an estimated ideal weight of 121–135 lbs. (with clothing and shoes) using Metropolitan norms. If her current weight is 145 lbs., then she is 17 lbs. overweight or approximately 13% overweight. A cutoff of 20% overweight is the accepted criterion for obesity as the associated health risks begin to increase significantly at this point.

While this normative approach is adequate for group comparisons in which only gross estimates of body composition are required, it is generally considered to be a very imprecise method for assessing adiposity. Individual differences in lean body mass (i.e., skeletal and muscle mass) can contribute to considerable variability in relative weight measures (Pyle, Mitchell, & Eckert, 1986). Furthermore, in cases where weight change is required, it is important to know to what degree weight change is attributable to changes in lean body mass versus changes in fat content. For example, weight loss in overweight individuals resulting primarily from muscle tissue and/or water loss can be more detrimental to those individuals than no weight loss at all (Garrow, 1986). Loss of lean body mass is particularly negative in dieters since this tissue accounts for 3 to 5 times more metabolic activity than fat tissue. Therefore, many researchers and clinicians are finding it necessary to use more precise estimates of body fat than relative weight. The following section describes these methods.

Estimates of Body Composition

Many measures of body fat have been developed over the past 40 years. These methods range widely in complexity and ease of administration. Formulae which use height and weight measures (i.e., body mass indexes) for estimation of body fat are the simplest methods. In addition to indexes of body mass, there are a variety of more direct procedures for estimating body composition, particularly as it relates to the content of fat in the body. The most common of these procedures is skinfold measurements. Underwater weighing, electrical impedance techniques, measurement of total body water, and measurement of total body potassium can also be used to estimate body fat percentage. However, discussion will be limited to the use of body mass indexes and skinfold measurements since these other methods are much more complex and expensive, and are therefore impractical for most clinical settings. Furthermore, the additional information offered by these techniques is not in proportion to their added expense and complexity.

Height/Weight Ratios. Weight/Height, Weight/(Height)^2, and Height/Weight$^{1/3}$ are the three height/weight ratios most commonly used. Billewicz, Kemsley, and Thomson (1962) compared these three indexes with relative adiposity as determined from body density measurements and concluded that Weight/(Height)^2 was the most valid estimate of body fat. This formula is often referred to as Quetelet's Body Mass Index (BMI) and it is computed by dividing the weight, *in kilograms,* by the square of the height, *in meters.* For men and women over 18 years of age, a BMI of 20 to 25 signifies the least threat of death or disease (Garrow, 1983). Guidelines for classifying individuals based on BMI vary somewhat, however, BMI ranges can be roughly designated as shown in Table 3.1.

Beumont, Al-Alami, and Touyz (1988) suggested that, in combination with other historical and clinical data, a BMI value of 16 or lower can be a very useful criterion for diagnosing anorexia nervosa.

From a practical standpoint, Quetelet's BMI is very appealing. It is easy to apply and it provides a measure that has been found to be highly correlated ($r = .96$) with the weight of fat in the body as estimated by body density, total body water, and total potassium (Webster, Hesp, & Garrow, 1984).

Skinfold Measurement. Of the various skinfold measurement techniques, the triceps and subscapular skinfolds are the most easily applied. They

Table 3.1. Body Mass Index

BMI	Weight Level
below 18	Severe underweight
18–20	Low weight
20–25	Normal weight
25–30	Overweight
30–40	Moderately obese
over 40	Grossly obese

have a high degree of reproducibility, and yield a degree of accuracy sufficient for most clinical and research purposes.

Triceps skinfold measurement is taken on the back of the arm midway between the point of the acromion (outer tip of shoulder) and olecranon process (lower tip of elbow with arm bent at a 90° angle). The subject is measured standing with the arm hanging loosely by his or her side. A fold of skin and subcutaneous tissue is then pinched between the thumb and forefinger at a distance of 1 cm above the site where the measurement is to be taken. The pressure on the fold should be exerted by the calipers. For increased reliability, at least two measures should be taken and averaged.

The subscapular skinfolds site is located approximately 1 cm below the bottom tip of the scapula (shoulder blade). Measurement is conducted by pinching the skin just inferior and lateral to the bottom tip of the scapula (along its vertebral border), resulting in a skinfold that is approximately 45° to the horizontal plane in the natural cleavage lines of the skin. Caliper measurement should be conducted similarly to that described for the triceps skinfold measurement and multiple readings should be taken to calculate an average value.

Data collected by the National Center for Health Statistics (1972–1973) has been analyzed by Cronk and Roche (1982) to develop race- and sex-specific reference tables for triceps and subscapular skinfolds. Table 3.2 lists percent body fat conversions for the sum of triceps and subscapular skinfold measurements. These converstions were calculated using data collected by Durnin and Womersley (1974) and can be used for both males, ages 17–72, and females, ages 16–68.

In using this table, one should add the obtained averages for the triceps and subscapular skinfolds and round this figure approximately to obtain the reference value in Table 3.2. For example, a 21-year-old woman with an average triceps skinfold of 6.6 mm and an average subscapular skinfold of 8.1 mm would have a sum of the two values equaling 14.7 mm. Using Table 3.2, this figure would be rounded to 20 mm. By moving across the row for a 20 mm sum of skinfolds to the reference column for

Table 3.2. Conversion of Skinfold Measurement to Percent Body Fat*
(Sum of Triceps and Subscapular Skinfolds)

Sum of Skinfolds (mm)	Males (age in years)				Females (age in years)			
	17–29	30–39	40–49	50+	16–29	30–39	40–49	50+
5	2.6	7.2	0.8	1.1	2.0	4.9	8.9	7.1
10	6.2	13.4	10.6	11.1	11.4	13.6	17.2	16.8
15	11.5	17.2	16.4	17.2	17.1	18.9	22.2	22.6
20	15.4	19.8	19.8	21.6	20.7	22.7	25.8	26.8
25	18.5	21.9	24.1	25.1	24.1	25.7	28.6	30.1
30	21.0	23.7	26.9	28.0	26.9	28.2	31.0	32.9
35	23.1	25.2	29.2	30.4	29.3	30.3	33.0	35.2
40	24.9	26.4	31.3	32.6	31.4	32.1	34.7	37.3
45	26.5	27.6	33.2	34.5	33.3	33.8	36.2	39.1
50	28.0	28.6	34.9	36.3	35.0	35.3	37.6	40.8
55	29.4	29.5	36.4	37.8	36.5	36.6	38.9	42.3
60	30.6	30.4	37.8	39.3	37.9	37.8	40.1	43.6
65	31.7	31.2	40.6	39.2	39.2	40.0	41.1	44.9
70	32.8	31.9	40.3	41.9	40.4	40.0	42.1	46.1
75	33.8	32.6	41.4	43.0	41.6	41.0	43.1	47.2
80	34.7	33.2	42.5	44.1	42.6	42.0	43.9	48.2
85	35.6	33.8	43.4	45.2	42.6	42.8	44.8	49.2
90	36.4	34.4	44.4	46.1	44.6	43.7	45.5	50.2
95	37.2	34.9	45.3	47.1	45.5	44.5	46.3	51.0
100	37.9	35.4	46.1	47.9	46.3	45.2	47.0	51.9
105	38.6	35.9	47.0	48.8	47.2	45.9	47.7	52.7
110	39.3	36.4	47.7	49.6	47.9	46.6	48.3	53.4
115	40.0	36.8	48.5	50.4	48.7	47.3	48.9	54.2
120	40.6	37.3	49.2	51.1	49.4	47.9	49.5	54.9

*Adapted from Durnin & Womersley, 1974

a 21-year-old female, one can see that this patient has about 20.7% body fat. The average body fat percentage is between 30% and 35% for women and between 25% and 30% for men. Below 20% body fat for women and 15% for men is considered very low and is usually characteristic of only highly athletic individuals. Many women will cease to menstruate if their body fat content falls below 15%. High body fat content is 30% to 35% for men and 35% to 40% for women while body fat content in excess of 35% and 40% is considered to represent obesity for men and women, respectively.

Clinical Implications of Adipose Morphology

Morphologic studies of adipose tissue have led researchers to postulate two subtypes of obesity (Hirsch & Knittle, 1970; Sjostrom & Bjorntorp, 1974). Early-onset obesity is characterized by an elevated fat cell number (hyperplastic obesity), and adult-onset obesity is associated with an increased fat cell size (hypertrophic obesity). While it is generally thought that hyperplastic obesity results from overfeeding during early stages of human development, there is some evidence which indicates that this pattern of obesity may be genetically influenced (Foch & McClearn, 1980). It is also generally assumed that the number of adipose cells is fixed by a certain age. However, some obesity research with experimental animals suggests that increases in fat cell number may occur at any point in life (Johnson & Hirsch, 1972; Bjorntorp, Karlsson, Gustafsson, Smith, Sjostrom, Cigolini, Storck, & Pettersson, 1979).

Clinically, both subtypes of obese individuals are able to achieve a significant amount of weight loss following dietary reduction. However, evidence from general clinical observations and empirical research suggests that individuals characterized by early-onset obesity are more likely to regain weight that has been lost. Krotkiewski, Sjostrom, Bjorntorp, Carlgren, Garellick, and Smith (1977) studied 100 obese women treated in an outpatient program using a 1100 kcal diet. They found that elevated fat cell number was associated with a rapid initial decrease in weight and a short duration at the reduced weight before regaining weight loss. On the other hand, expanded fat cell size without fat cell hyperplasia was associated with a slower weight loss, but a longer duration of reduced weight prior to relapse. The tendency to relapse in hyperplastic obese individuals may be related to the irreversibility of fat cell number. It has been proposed that fat cell size may influence energy balance in such a way as to increase the drive to eat with decreasing fat cell size (Bjorntorp, 1977). In hyperplastic obese individuals, the degree to which fat cells must be reduced to achieve adequate weight loss may produce a very difficult compensatory drive by the body to refill the adipocytes.

The techniques for measuring fat cell number and fat cell size are beyond the scope of this text. The interested reader may refer to Bjorntorp (1977) for more information on these techniques. However, research evidence supports the likelihood that early-onset obesity will be characterized by hyperplasia of fat cells, while adult-onset obesity will be associated with hypertrophic fat cells. Clinicians and researchers should be aware of these relationships and of their prognostic implications. Of particular importance is the fact that repeated weight cycling (i.e., weight loss and regain) leads to greater metabolic efficiency and, hence, greater difficulty in future weight loss or prevention of future weight gain (Foreyt, 1987). Thus, for individuals with early-onset obesity and a history of weight loss failures, it may be advisable to design treatment to achieve mild to moderate weight loss and acceptance of a body size that is somewhat larger than "normal."

SELF-MONITORING

Self-monitoring is one of the most widely used procedures in behavioral assessment of eating disorders. Self-monitoring data can be helpful for diagnosis, functional analysis, and evaluation of the efficacy of treatment procedures.

Self-monitoring of food consumption was an integral part of the early behavior modification programs for obesity and it continues to be emphasized in behavioral treatments today. Self-monitoring procedures generally instruct the patient to record such information as type and amount of foods consumed, mood before and after eating, hunger before and after eating, and environmental circumstances prior to and during eating. This information is used to analyze functional and caloric aspects of eating episodes, which can then be used in treatment.

A common finding is that negative affect is often an antecedent to binge eating and often precedes both binging and purging in bulimia nervosa patients (Schlundt, Johnson, & Jarrell, 1985, 1986; Johnson & Larson, 1982; Davis, Freeman, & Garner, 1988). Other factors associated with problematic eating include hunger, regularity of eating, activity prior to eating, time of day, and environmental setting. In general, obese and bulimic individuals are most likely to overeat or binge when they have skipped one or more meals during the day and are hungry. Often, they have recently encountered a distressing or boring situation and overeat when they are alone. Their binges typically occur in the afternoon following work or school, and in the evening or weekend hours when they are often alone and are feeling bored or depressed. Purging by bulimia nervosa patients can also be related to factors such as environmental stress regularity of eating. However, purging is often a function of the types of food consumed and, most importantly, if the meal was defined as a binge.

We have found that the assessment of naturalistic factors associated with eating are instrumental in providing effective treatment for persons with eating disorders. Thus, we have developed a fairly detailed self-monitoring procedure that patients are asked to utilize on a daily basis. Information regarding each individual eating episode is recorded on a separate page of a self-monitoring booklet provided to the patient. In addition to the amount and type of food and the variables mentioned above, a section for comments is provided on each page. Many patients report that it is helpful for them to write down what they are feeling at that time. For bulimia nervosa and purging anorexic patients, the self-monitoring form also includes a section to report the occurrence of purging, and mood and hunger associated with purging. However, as this section is not relevant for patients who do not evidence purgative behavior, we have alternative self-monitoring forms which do not include this section. An example of a typical self-monitoring record is provided in Figure. 3.5.

From this figure it can be seen that the patient ate dinner with her co-workers following work. Her mood just prior to eating was neutral and she was moderately hungry. She reports eating less than normal, that her mood was also neutral following eating, and that she was not hungry after eating. No purgative behavior took place. It is important to note that she ate 100% of the salad but only 25% of the fried chicken pattie. That she ate 100% of the chocolate yogurt is not very unusual for a restrictive eater because yogurt is often seen by these patients as a "safe," low-calorie food. She was aware that her eating was less than normal in amount and wrote in the comment section, "I don't know why except I was afraid to eat more." She also noted that she lost her appetite when she began to eat and that this was an unusual occurrence for her. Collectively, this information suggests that this patient is uncomfortable eating in front of her co-workers, especially when eating in a restaurant setting. She most likely eats slower, takes smaller bites, and worries about looking socially appropriate, all of which have the effect of stifling one's appetite. However, the problem with this behavior is that she is likely to feel deprived and is likely to experience a return of her appetite when she gets home. The risk for binge eating in such a state is significantly increased. The patient can be presented with this formulation of the eating episode and instructed how to alter her eating so that it is more consistent throughout the day and across different situations.

Patients are educated about the therapeutic benefits of self-monitoring and are instructed in the proper method to record food consumption. A frequent question that patients ask is how to define a binge. In general, behavioral treatment programs have employed a subjective definition of binge eating, that is, a feeling of having "overeaten," and recent data from our clinic have shown this definition to be reliable and valid.

Typically, we have patients monitor their food consumption for two weeks before entering therapy. This procedure accomplishes several things. It allows for the collection of naturalistic information to assist in making a diagnosis and case formulation (Williamson, Prather, Goreczny, Davis, & McKenzie, 1989), it provides baseline data for assessing treatment outcome, and it allows the patient time to receive feedback about performance in self-monitoring before treatment begins.

There are several aspects of the self-monitoring information that are most useful for examining treatment outcome. This information can be easily quantified using the information recorded in the self-monitoring books, and it can then be depicted in tabular form to aid in clearly docu-

DAY _Tues_ DATE _2-19_ TIME _6:00_ AM. **PM**

MEAL: Breakfast. Lunch. **Dinner** Snack

ACTIVITY PRIOR TO EATING:
Class. Exercise. Relaxation. Social. TV. **Work**
Other -

WITH WHOM: Alone. Date Spouse. Family. Friend.
Other - _Coworkers_

MEAL WAS EATEN WHERE:
Kitchen. **Dining Room** Restaurant. Work. Den. Bedroom.
Living Room. Other -

MOOD PRIOR TO EATING:
Very Positive. Positive. **Neutral** Negative. Very Negative.
Describe -

HUNGER PRIOR TO EATING:
Very Hungry. **Moderately Hungry** Neutral. Not Hungry. Full

AMOUNT EATEN:
Undereat Normal. Slight Overeat. Moderate Overeat. Binge

MOOD AFTER EATING:
Very Positive. Positive. **Neutral** Negative. Very Negative
Describe -

HUNGER AFTER EATING:
Very Hungry. Moderately Hungry. Neutral. **Not Hungry** Full

PURGE: Yes **No**
If Yes - Vomit. Laxatives or Diuretics
If Laxatives or Diuretics, how many? _____

TIME OF PURGE: _____ AM. PM

MOOD AFTER PURGING:
Very Positive. Positive. Neutral. Negative. Very Negative
Describe -

HUNGER AFTER PURGING:
Very Hungry. Moderately Hungry. Neutral. Not Hungry. Full

Accurate Description of Food or Drink Item	Amount
Salad - turkey, bacon & 1 tbsp dressing	100%
Rice w/mushroom	40%
Fried chicken pattie	25%
Carrots (1 cup)	50%
1 cup of choc yogurt	100%
Apple	40%

Comments: _Meal was good - I don't know why except I was afraid to eat more. Once I started eating I noticed I didn't have much of an appetite. That is unusual for me._

FIGURE 3.5. Example of self-monitoring record.

menting baseline parameters. Figure 3.6 illustrates an example of data which can be used for evaluating treatment outcome.

This figure represents two weeks of self-monitoring. In obtaining this information, all of the eating episodes for two weeks were added to yield a total number of eating episodes for the two weeks and an average number of eating episodes per day. In this figure those values are 40 and 2.9 respectively. Eating episodes are also categorized as to type. For example,

Food Monitoring Summary Sheet

Table represents ___2___ weeks of data.

EATING VARIABLES	Undereat	Normal	Slight Overeat	Moderate Overeat	Binge	Purge
NUMBER	2	15	10	5	8	10
HUNGER PRIOR [1]	1.6	2.4	3.3	3.1	3.8	1.0
HUNGER AFTER [1]	2.4	1.8	2.1	2.5	1.0	1.8
MOOD PRIOR [1]	2.6	3.2	2.9	2.6	3.9	4.6
MOOD AFTER [1]	2.1	3.1	3.2	3.8	4.8	2.6
AT HOME	0%	40%	50%	60%	75%	90%
AWAY FROM HOME	100%	60%	50%	40%	25%	10%
ALONE	0%	33%	40%	60%	88%	100%
WITH OTHERS	100%	66%	60%	40%	12%	0%
MORNING	0%	13%	10%	20%	12%	10%
AFTERNOON	50%	40%	30%	40%	25%	30%
EVENING	50%	47%	60%	40%	62%	60%

PURGES AFTER BINGING	100%
PURGES W/OUT BINGING	20%
TOTAL EATING EPISODES	40
TOTAL EPISODES PER DAY	2.9

[1] Average ratings of hunger and mood based on 5 pt. scale with 5 indicating greater hunger and more negative mood.

FIGURE 3.6. Self-monitoring summary record.

this figure shows the patient to have recorded 2 undereating episodes, 15 normal eating episodes, and so forth. The number of purges is also listed. For each type of eating episode, five major variables of eating are considered: hunger, mood, location, time, and with whom the meal was eaten. The patient's ratings of hunger and mood in the self-monitoring forms are assigned values from 1 to 5 with 1 representing being full and very positive in mood and 5 representing being very hungry and very negative in mood. These ratings are then averaged and rounded to one decimal place. In this figure the patient recorded 8 binge-eating episodes, an average hunger prior to binging of 3.8 (i.e., approximately very hungry) and an average hunger after eating of 1.0 (i.e., full). Mood before and after binging was found to average 3.9 and 4.8 respectively, which indicates a negative mood associated with binge eating. This figure also shows that the patient experienced 75% or 6 of the 8 binges at home and 25% or 2 of the 8 binges away from home. Eighty-eight percent of the binge episodes occurred when the patient was alone and 12% occurred with other people present. Only 12% of the patient's binges took place during the morning hours while 25% and 62% occurred in the afternoon and evening hours respectively. This type of information has also been calculated for each of the other types of eating episodes and for purges. Finally, percentages are calculated for the number of purge episodes that occurred after binging and for those that occurred in the absence of binging. This figure shows that purging followed binging 100% of the time, but that the patient purged 20% of the time even though she did not indicate a prior binge.

Recording self-monitoring data in this way allows one to examine the functional relationships among the variables. For example, examination of the data in Figure 3.5 shows that this patient frequently binges when very hungry and very negative in mood. Also, binges are associated with being alone, being at home, and evening hours. Based on this information, treatment for binge eating should target the following: (1) reduction of time spent alone by the patient, (2) elimination of severe dietary restriction so that the patient is never extremely hungry, and (3) training of problem-solving skills to reduce the severity and frequency of negative mood states. In a similar manner, the variables associated with purging can be targeted for change and those associated with normal eating can be reinforced. The following case example illustrates how self-monitoring data can be used for diagnosis, case formulation, and establishment of baseline data.

Case Example. John was a 38-year-old unmarried businessman who presented at the clinic complaining of excessive weight gain. He reported that during the past 5 years he had become less active and had gradually gained about 50 lbs. In addition to a standard interview and testing protocol for the assessment of eating disorders, John was asked to monitor his food consumption in the manner described previously. Examination of John's self-monitoring over a two-week period showed that he binged approximately three times per week, frequently following a stressful day at work. In addition, John generally ate very small meals for breakfast and lunch, and then ate a comparatively large meal in the evening. Although John did not typically record this evening meal as a binge, he did indicate recurrent small snacking episodes during the evening hours following this meal, which he considered to be excessive. Finally, the majority of John's eating episodes occurred in either the living room in front of the television or in the bedroom while working at his desk.

From this information and that obtained through interview and testing, it was determined that John did not meet the criteria for bulimia nervosa as he did not evidence purgative behavior or extreme methods to lose or control weight (e.g., severe dietary restriction, starvation, extreme exercise). He did report depression and self-deprecating thoughts following binge eating and was aware that his eating pattern was abnormal. Thus, he was given the diagnosis of compulsive overeating. In formulating John's case, the self-monitoring data were examined to pinpoint the problem areas in his eating behavior. John apparently developed the habit of restricting his dietary intake during the day, which left him very hungry during the evening when he was at home alone. He also ate many of his meals in places other than at the dining room table. This practice has been found to cause sensations of hunger to become associated with numerous activities and settings (e.g., watching television). It was concluded that John's pattern of eating precipitated compulsive overeating in the evening hours and binge eating following stressful days. This eating style combined with a reduction in physical activity was sufficient to cause significant weight gain. John was informed of these observations and instructed in behavior modification techniques to reduce the tendency to eat compulsively and binge eat. He was also placed on a program of regular but moderate exercise. The weekly average of binge episodes and overeating episodes from this self-monitoring data was used to establish a baseline from which to judge treatment efficacy.

Probably the biggest problem with self-monitoring procedures is that they require effort and continuous commitment to recording eating behavior. Patient compliance with record keeping tends to be poor because of these requirements. However, we have found that there are several steps which can be taken to increase patient compliance. These steps include: (a) thorough instruction in the proper self-monitoring technique and explanation of its therapeutic use, (b) sharing with the patient the relationship between therapeutic recommendations and functional analysis of self-monitoring records, and (c) periodic feedback of progress in behavior change which is derived from self-monitoring data.

Summary

As described in the sections above, the use of behavioral assessment techniques can provide unique and very valuable information about eating behavior and body composition. Test meals have been used to analyze psychological and behavioral correlates of both normal and binge eating in the laboratory, and have been instrumental in developing treatment techniques. In addition, test meals can be employed to assess treatment efficacy both during and following the treatment period.

Accurate measurement of weight and body composition is crucial to providing adequate treatment to those with eating disorders. The use of weight tables to determine the percentage difference of an individual's weight from an ideal weight is frequently employed. While this normative approach may be adequate for conducting group comparisons, it is not sufficiently accurate for usage in clinical work or research with individuals. It is recommended that one use either the Body Mass Index (BMI) or skinfold measurement technique for these purposes.

Lastly, self-monitoring has long been utilized in treatment programs for eating disorders. The use of self-monitoring data can be used to conduct a functional analysis of a patient's eating behavior so that the situational and emotional antecedents and consequences of eating can be targeted during treatment.

Chapter 4
✗ Body Image Assessment

As noted in Chapter 1, body image disturbances have been implicated in the etiology and maintenance of anorexia and bulimia nervosa. Despite years of research and discussion by clinical researchers, the definition of this construct is still far from clear. A wide range of phenomena have been investigated under the rubric of "body image." For example, body image has been conceptualized as the picture of our own body which we form in our mind (Schilder, 1935), a neural representation of bodily experience (Head, 1920), the feelings we have about our bodies (Secord & Jourard, 1953), and a personality construct (Fisher & Cleveland, 1958). More recently, Garner and Garfinkel (1981) described body image disturbance as a two-part phenomenon, including a "perceptual" component as well as an affective or cognitive component. The latter has also been referred to as "body image dissatisfaction." Williamson, Davis, Goreczny, and Blouin (1989) have described a third type of body image disturbance which they termed "preference for thinness."

The recent revision of DSM-III (American Psychiatric Association, 1987) has recognized symptoms of body image disturbances to be essential characteristics of anorexia and bulimia nervosa. The diagnostic criteria for anorexia nervosa include body image *distortion* (e.g., claiming to "feel fat" even when emaciated), a *weight phobia* (e.g., intense fear of gaining weight or becoming fat), and a *preference for thinness* (e.g., refusal to maintain normal body weight). The diagnostic criteria for bulimia nervosa include a "persistent overconcern with body shape and weight," suggesting that body image disturbances are symptomatic of bulimia nervosa as well. Thus, measurement of body image disturbances is essential for comprehensive evaluation of these disorders.

A number of measurement techniques have been developed to assess body image distortion. The most commonly used approaches have been

(a) distorting image techniques, (b) body-part size estimation, and (c) silhouettes of differing body sizes. In addition, a variety of attitudinal measures have been developed to measure dissatisfaction with body size. This chapter will discuss our conceptualization of body image and will review methods for assessing disturbances of body image.

THE CONSTRUCT OF BODY IMAGE

Earlier research treated body image as a unitary construct. This approach led to very little progress in defining and understanding the phenomenon. Recent research on body image has attempted to identify and analyze the components of body image disturbance. The following sections review three components of body image which have been combined to form a new theoretical model of body image. These elements of body image and the theoretical model are described in the following sections.

Body Size Distortion

Body size distortion is generally conceptualized as a phenomenon involving the perception of one's current body size. Methods for assessing body image disturbance usually require subjects to indicate their perception of body size which is then compared to actual body size measurements to determine a person's perceptual accuracy. Using these techniques, body size distortion is measured as a function of the degree to which the person misperceives actual body size. Anorexics and bulimics have often been found to overestimate actual body size and thus evidence body size distortion in the sense of seeing themselves as "fat" even when they are thin. Body size distortion has been investigated via body-part size estimation, distorting image methods, and silhouettes of female body sizes.

Preference for Thinness

Preference for thinness has received only limited attention as a type of body image disturbance (Williamson, Davis, Goreczny, Bennett, & Gleaves, in press). Preference for thinness may be conceptualized as an individual's "ideal body size," or a body size which is used as an ideal standard for judging satisfaction with current body size. Research related to this construct suggests that individuals who intensely fear weight gain (e.g., anorexics and bulimics) prefer a body size which is significantly thinner than those who do not have such fears. Thus, it is proposed that a strong preference for thinness should be inversely related to a fear of fatness. The primary effect of preferring an extremely thin body size is that it drives behavior to achieve thinness and increases dissatisfaction with body size, as discussed in the next section. Methodology for assessing preference for thinness has generally involved measuring the subject's selection of an ideal body size.

Body Size Dissatisfaction

Body size dissatisfaction typically has been investigated using attitudinal measures. A number of studies have utilized questionnaires as a means of measuring dissatisfaction with body size (Garner, Olmstead, Polivy, & Garfinkel, 1983; Johnson, Lewis, Love, Lewis, & Stuckey, 1984; Katzman & Wolchik, 1984; Leon, Lucas, Colligan, Ferdinande, & Kamp, 1985). More recently, however, the discrepancy between actual body size estimates and ideal body size estimates has been used to derive an index of body size dissatisfaction (Williamson, Davis, Goreczny, & Blouin, 1989). For example, a large discrepancy between perceived body size and ideal body size would be indicative of extreme dissatisfaction whereas a small discrepancy would indicate a slight dissatisfaction. Williamson, Davis, et al. (in press) have proposed that body image distortion may interact with intense preference for thinness to produce extreme body size dissatisfaction in some normal weight persons (e.g., bulimia nervosa).

Theoretical Model of Body Image Disturbance

We have developed a theoretical model of body image disturbances which delineates how body image distortion, preference for thinness, and body size dissatisfaction interact with fear of fatness to produce static and dynamic disturbances of body image. The theoretical model, illustrated in Figure 4.1, proposes that body size dissatisfaction is a function of both body size distortion and preference for thinness. Body size distortion is conceptualized as the degree of perceptual accuracy of current body size (CBS). As noted earlier, anorexics and bulimics have been found to overestimate actual body size. Preference for thinness is conceptualized as the degree to which a person prefers an ideal body size (IBS) which is thinner than that of others of similar size. The degree of dissatisfaction with body size is determined by the degree of distortion, preference for thinness, or both. As CBS increases (body size distortion) and IBS decreases (preference for thinness), body size dissatisfaction increases. The theoretical model proposes that body size dissatisfaction is not a static phenomenon.

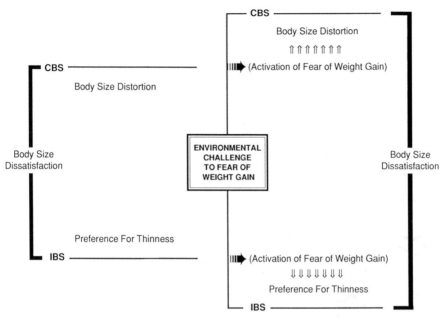

FIGURE 4.1. Model of body image disturbances.

Instead, body image disturbance is thought to be influenced by environmental stimuli which may affect body size distortion and/or preference for thinness by activating an individual's fear of weight gain. Figure 4.1 illustrates this theoretical model. The left side of the figure depicts a baseline level of body size dissatisfaction typically seen in anorexia or bulimia nervosa. The degree of body dissatisfaction is dependent upon the person's CBS and IBS estimates. The right side of Figure 4.1 illustrates the reactive effects of body image disturbance when environmental events activate fear of weight gain. Body size dissatisfaction is increased as a result of an increase in body size distortion or a stronger preference for thinness, or both. Environmental challenges, such as eating or weighing "too much," or wearing tight clothing, are hypothesized to activate fear of weight gain which, in turn, worsens body size distortion and/or preference for thinness. Normal weight females without an eating disorder would be predicted to have less body size distortion (indicated by a smaller current body size estimate) and less preference for thinness (indicated by a larger ideal body size estimate), as well as less fear of weight gain. Thus, persons of normal weight without an eating disorder would be predicted to have less static body size dissatisfaction and be less reactive to environmental challenges. The following case examples illustrate how environmental stimuli may differentially affect the body image disturbance of anorexic and bulimic patients.

Case Example. Beth was a 21-year-old art student who presented for treatment of bulimia nervosa. She had been dissatisfied with her body size since age 14 and by age 17 was unable to eat any foods, except those very low in calories, without purging via self-induced vomiting. Beth was 5 ft. 4 in. tall and weighed 121 lbs. Although she did not view herself as larger than other females of her same height and weight, she wanted to be very thin. Beth would become very upset after eating, stating that she felt like a "hippo." She refused to be weighed on days she had eaten over 500 calories and often refused to go to school on days where she had eaten a normal breakfast. Careful evauation of Beth's body image disturbance indicated that the act of eating caused distortion of current body size which produced a high degree of body size dissatisfaction. The act of eating served to worsen Beth's body image disturbance by challenging her fear of weight gain. This information proved valuable in Beth's treatment plan as desensitization of emotional reactions to stomach distension after eating led to decreased dissatisfaction with body size.

Case Example. Donna was an 18-year-old freshman who weighed 92 lbs. at 4 ft., 10 in. She presented for treatment of bulimia nervosa. She reported frequent episodes of binge eating, which were followed by vigorous exercise, such as two hours of running. When Donna presented for treatment she was running after every meal or snack. Although Donna viewed her body size as "a bit too small" she was very afraid of gaining weight. She stated that each time she ate she began to fear possible weight gain and would feel an urge to run until she had burned off the calories. She denied feeling any larger after eating, but was unable to control her fears of getting fat. Thus, the act of eating served to activate Donna's fear of weight gain which led to an increase in preference for thinness and an increase in body size dissatisfaction. With treatment, Donna learned that moderate eating did not produce weight gain and that she did not need to continue losing weight to avoid being fat.

Case Example. Julie was a 22-year-old college student who was referred for treatment of anorexia nervosa. She was 5 ft., 2 in. tall and weighed 78 lbs. Although she previously had weighed as much as 102 lbs., Julie denied any active attempts to diet or lose weight. Self-induced vomiting and laxative abuse were also denied. Julie did admit to daily exercise, but denied feeling like her activity level was excessive. Eating patterns were described as "healthy," but were judged to be very restrictive by the clinician. Body size dissatisfaction was not present as Julie viewed herself as very thin and showed no preference for a thinner body size. In other words, Julie did not prefer to be smaller than she was at the time of presentation, and thus was not dissatisfied with her body size.

Due to her low body weight and restrictive eating pattern, Julie was treated via cognitive-behavioral treatment for anorexia. Emphasis was placed on appropriate meal planning and consumption of "forbidden" foods. Julie was placed on a weight gain treatment program and gained approximately 3 lbs. during her first week of treatment. She reported feeling good about eating a variety of foods and she exhibited few, if any, overt signs of distress.

By the end of the third week of treatment, however, Julie had gained 7 lbs. and she began to exhibit signs of extreme dissatisfaction with her body size. She perceived herself to be much larger than she had prior to treatment. Her preference for thinness had also increased causing an even greater discrepancy between her perceived current size and her ideal size. Julie began resisting treatment, by hiding food, as her fear of weight gain increased. As treatment continued a greater emphasis was placed on disturbances of body image. In particular, body image therapy was used as a treatment of strategy to decrease Julie's fears related to the changes in her body.

Empirical Support for the Model

The model proposes that, as a group, anorexics and bulimics should be characterized by body image distortion and/or preference for thinness, resulting in greater body size dissatisfaction than occurs in normals of similar body size. Support for this prediction is somewhat mixed (Cash & Brown, 1987) in that some studies have found evidence for body image disturbances in these eating disorders and others have not. This research will be summarized in the following sections which discuss the various methods for assessing body image.

A few studies have investigated changes in body image following challenges to fears of weight gain. Across a variety of environmental stimuli (eating, weighing, mirror confrontation), worsening of body image distortion has been found in both bulimics and anorexics with body-part size estimation tasks, but not with distorting image techniques. Although the effects of environmental challenges on body image *distortion* have been demonstrated with at least one type of methodology, investigations of body image reactivity in terms of body size dissatisfaction and preference for thinness have not been conducted. Therefore, support for the theoretical model is strongest for predictions related to static body image disturbances in anorexia and bulimia nervosa. Further research on the factors that determine dynamic changes in body image are now needed.

The theoretical model presented in Figure 4.1 also explains body size dissatisfaction associated with obesity. The theory proposes that body size dissatisfaction is caused by a discrepancy between current body size and ideal body size. The body size of obese patients is very large and thus the perception of this discrepancy is realistic, and not distorted. Dissatisfaction is predicted because the individual prefers to be thinner.

MEASUREMENT OF BODY IMAGE

The following sections will describe the most commonly used assessment techniques in the measurement of body image disturbance. Reliability and validity data will be provided when available. Specific detail will be provided for the Body Image Assessment procedure (BIA; Williamson et al., 1985) as this technique is easily administered and has been used extensively with eating disorder patients.

Distorting Image Techniques

Distorting image techniques require subjects to estimate their overall body size using images of their own bodies, such as in a mirror or a camera. An "adjustable body-distorting mirror," which could be bent by the subject to provide distorted images of subjects, was the first of these measures to be developed (Traub & Orbach, 1964). A similar procedure, the Distorting Photograph Technique (DPT; Glucksman & Hirsch, 1969) was developed several years later. This technique used a variable, anamorphic lens that was capable of distorting a standard slide photograph of a subject by 20% over or under the original size of the slide. More recently, the Video Distortion Technique (VDT; Allebeck, Hallberg, & Espmark, 1976) was developed. This procedure involved a modified television camera that could electronically distort the subject's image to be smaller or larger than the actual size. With each of these measurement techniques, subjects are required to adjust the image to match their perceived actual size and often their ideal size. The degree of adjustment is typically used as a measure of body image *distortion*.

Temporal stability of distorting image techniques has been demonstrated over one to three weeks (Freeman, Thomas, Solyom, & Hunter, 1984; Garfinkel, Moldofsky, Garner, Stancer, & Coscina, 1978) as well as over one year (Garfinkel, Moldofsky, & Garner, 1979). By correlating profile and frontal body image scores, Freeman et al. (1984) obtained satisfactory internal consistency estimates for the video distortion technique.

With regard to discriminant validity, three controlled studies using distorting image techniques have shown anorexic subjects to overestimate their body size to a greater degree than control subjects (Freeman, Thomas, Solyom, & Miles, 1983; Garfinkel et al., 1978; Wingate & Christie, 1978). However, three other controlled studies reported no differences between anorexics' estimates of body size and those of controls (Freeman, Thomas, Solyom, & Koopman, 1985; Garfinkel, Moldofsky, & Garner, 1979; Touyz, Beumont, Collins, McCabe, & Jupp, 1984). Bulimic subjects, on the other hand, have been shown to consistently overestimate their body size in two studies using distorting image techniques (Freeman et al., 1985; Touyz, Beumont, Collins, & Cowie, 1985). It is of interest to note that these two studies also compared body size overestimation of anorexics and bulimics, as well as controls. Freeman et al. (1985) reported that bulimics with a history of anorexia overestimated body size more than anorexic subjects and bulimics without a history of anorexia. Touyz et al. (1985) found that 95% of bulimics overestimated body size compared to only 48% of anorexics. Seime, Wiener, and Fremouw (1988) utilized a video distortion camera in the investigation of body image disturbance with clinical bulimics, subjects identified as "high risk" for bulimia, and subjects identified as "low risk" for bulimia. They found that clinical subjects viewed themselves at 105% of their actual body size and selected an ideal body size which was 81% of their actual size. High risk subjects viewed themselves at 115% of their actual body size with ideal size selection of 83% actual body size. The low risk subjects viewed themselves at 100% of their actual size (accurate perception), but still chose an ideal body size slightly smaller than their actual size (95%).

Concurrent validity of a modified VDT procedure was investigated by Freeman and his colleagues (Freeman et al., 1984). Body image distortion was found to be moderately correlated with the EAT (Garner & Garfinkel, 1979) and body image dissatisfaction (derived by subtracting ideal image from perceived image) was moderately correlated with measures of depression.

In summary, distorting image techniques have been shown to be reliable and internally consistent. By using these techniques body image distortion has been consistently demonstrated in bulimia nervosa patients but less consistently in anorexia nervosa. By using this methodology, individuals at "high risk" for bulimia have also been shown to overestimate their body size and prefer a smaller size. However, distorting image techniques have not proven useful in the measurement of environmental reactivity of body image disturbance as they appear to be insensitive to dynamic variations in body image over time.

Body-Part Size Estimation

The first of these techniques, the "movable caliper technique" or Visual Size Estimation task (VSE), was developed by Reitman and Cleveland (1964). It was later adapted for use with anorexic populations by Slade and Russell (1973). This system uses two lights mounted in tracks on a horizontal bar. A pulley allows for the symmetrical movement of the two lights which are adjusted by the subject to estimate the width or depth of specific body regions. Slade and Russell (1973) introduced a statistical definition of body perception accuracy called the Body Perception Index (BPI). Accuracy of each body region is derived using the formula BPI = perceived size/axctual size $\times$ 100. Actual size is determined with the use of an anthropometer or body caliper. The BPIs for each body area are often averaged to determine a composite index of body perception accuracy.

Ruff and Barrios (1986) recently introduced a size estimation technique known as the Body Image Detection Device (BIDD) that consists of a standard overhead projector which is manipulated to allow a 1 cm wide horizontal band of light to be projected on the wall. Two posterboard templates, one in the shape of a triangle, and the other with a triangle removed from it, are moved through wooden guides mounted to the top of the projector, allowing for the horizontal width of the band of light to expand or converge. The subject is asked to adjust the band of light to estimate the widths of various body parts. A modification of the BIDD has been introduced more recently (Thompson, J. K. & Thompson, C. M., 1986), which allows for the simultaneous presentation of four horizontal beams of light, so that size estimations of four body regions may be obtained during one trial.

Internal consistency and temporal stability have been demonstrated for the body-part size estimation techniques (Pierloot & Houben, 1978; Strober, Goldenberg, Green, & Saxon, 1979; Ruff & Barrios, 1986). With regard to discriminant validity, anorexic subjects have been shown to overestimate body size to a greater degree than controls in three controlled studies (Pierloot & Houben, 1978; Slade, 1977; Slade & Russell, 1973), although six studies have reported no differences between anorexics and controls (Ben-Tovim & Crisp, 1984; Button, Fransella, & Slade, 1977; Casper, Halmi, Goldberg, Eckert, & Davis, 1979; Crisp & Kalucy, 1974; Norris, 1984; Strober et al., 1979). Results of body-part size estimation studies with bulimics have also produced mixed results with two studies reporting greater overestimation of body size by bulimic subjects than controls (Ruff & Barrios, 1986; Willmuth, Leitenberg, Rosen, Fondacaro, & Gross, 1985) and two studies reporting no differences between bulimics and controls (Birtchnell, Lacey, & Harte, 1985; Norris, 1984).

In summary, body-part size estimation procedures have been shown to be reliable and internally consistent. However, degree of overestimation has been inconsistent with both anorexics and bulimics. Further investigation of the validity of these techniques is needed before they can be used confidently for assessing eating disorder patients.

Attitudinal Measures

A number of questionnaires have been used to assess attitudinal components of body size dissatisfaction. The Body Cathexis Scale (Secord & Jourard, 1953) was one of the earliest self-report inventories designed to assess satisfaction with body size. The scale consists of 46 questions related to body parts and functions, such as hair and energy level. Each item is rated from 1 (have strong feelings and wish change could somehow be made) to 5 (consider myself fortunate) on the basis of how one feels about each body part or function. The authors reported internal consistency estimates of .78 and .83 for males and females, respectively. In addition, moderate correlations have been found between the body cathexis scale and the self-cathexis scale, indicating that feelings about the body are commensurate with feelings about the self, when both are appraised by similar scales (Secord & Jourard, 1953).

The Body-Self Relations Questionnaire (BSRQ; Winstead & Cash, 1984) has 140 items to which the individual responds on a 5-point Likert scale ranging from definitely agree to definitely disagree. The items concern the person's attitudes and actions toward three somatic domains (physical appearance, physical fitness, and physical health).

The Body Dissatisfaction Scale of the EDI (Garner, Olmstead, & Polivy, 1983) has been used for the assessment of body size dissatisfaction. This scale has nine items which reflect the belief that specific body parts associated with shape change or increased "fatness" at puberty are too large. The authors reported item-total correlations ranging from .50 to .83. Cronbach's alpha correlations of .90 and .91 were found, indicating a high degree of internal consistency. In addition, concurrent validity has been shown, correlating the Body Dissatisfaction Scale with other scales designed to measure body dissatisfaction (Berscheid, Walster, & Bohrnstedt, 1973).

In a recent review, Cash and Brown (1987) concluded that all controlled studies of body image disturbance which included an attitudinal measure reported greater body size dissatisfaction in eating disorder groups than in controls. The BSRQ and Body Dissatisfaction Scale have been most fully developed from the perspective of adequate psychometrics.

Computerized Assessment

Schlundt and Bell (1988) have developed a microcomputer program for assessing cognitive and affective components of body image called the Body Image Testing System (BITS). The program is written in TURBO PASCAL language for IBM-PC and compatible systems which use interactive computer graphics. The program generates frontal view and side view silhouettes of a human body. Subjects can make the body silhouette image grow smaller or larger for nine independent body regions (face, neck, shoulders, chest, arms, breasts, stomach, hips, and thighs) via the computer control system. The procedure allows for minute adjustments for specific body areas. Subjects are instructed to adjust the figure to their perceived "actual" size, their "ideal" size, or how fat or thin their body "feels."

Schlundt and Bell (1988) found that most college-aged women were not satisfied with their bodies and that a greater degree of dissatisfaction was associated with the stomach, hips, and thighs. Actual-ideal differences were correlated with degree of overweight. The authors have developed a perceptual distortion measure by taking the difference between actual body size scores and scores predicted from height, weight, and degree of overweight. Obese women showed greater overall perceptual distortion (compared to college-aged women) and relatively higher distortion of the stomach and thighs. Validity was tested by correlating the actual-ideal discrepancy scores with the perceptual scores and a wide variety of measures that reflect body dissatisfaction and disordered eating behavior. The actual-ideal discrepancy was moderately correlated with all other measures for the college-aged women although less so for obese women. Fewer significant correlations were obtained with regard to the perceptual distortion measure, however, for both college-aged women and obese women.

The BITS is very easy to administer and preliminary data suggest that it has promise as a measure of body image characteristics. Clinical research using bulimia and anorexia nervosa subjects is now needed. Presently the BITS must be regarded as a promising experimental procedure in the early stage of development.

Silhouettes

Gottesman and Caldwell (1966) first developed a series of silhouettes of body size as a projective measure of body image. A type of individualized silhouette methodology was also used by Counts and Adams (1985). Each subject was presented with a set of seven silhouettes, one having been drawn from the subject's actual photograph and the remaining silhouettes representing 2.5, 5, and 7.5% increases and decreases in the size of certain body areas of the original figure. Subjects were asked to select both their actual size and their ideal size.

Williamson et al. (1985) introduced a new method for measuring body image disturbances called the Body Image Assessment (BIA) procedure. This method is quite simple in that it involves selection of a silhouette of a female body which most closely resembles the subject's perception of her current body size (CBS) and ideal body size (IBS). Specifically, the procedure requires the use of nine body image cards, 6 in. × 4 in. (15.4 cm × 10.3 cm) which are depicted in Figure 4.2. On each card there is a drawing of a female figure whose body ranges from very thin to very obese, in incremental steps. The procedure for administering the body image assessment is to place the cards in a random order on a table in front of the subject. The subject is then given the following instructions: "Select the card that most accurately depicts your current body size, as you perceive it to be. Please be honest. You must choose only one card and you may not rearrange the cards to directly compare them." After the subject chooses a card, the experimenter records the card number (which is written on the back of each card). The cards are reshuffled and again are presented in random order. The subject is given these instructions: "Please select the card that most accurately depicts the body size that you would most prefer. Again, be honest and do not rearrange the cards." Once the subject chooses a card, the experimenter records the card number. The entire procedure generally requires less than 1 minute. From these data, one can derive current body size (CBS) and ideal body size (IBS) scores for each subject. The difference between the two scores (current minus ideal) yields a body size dissatisfaction score.

Previous research has shown that weight is positively correlated with both CBS (.70) and IBS (.33). Therefore, consideration of actual body size

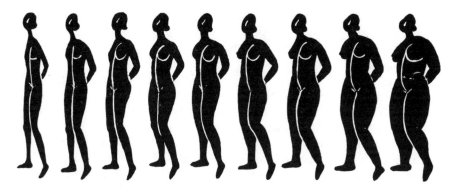

FIGURE 4.2. Body size silhouette for Body Image Assessment.

dimensions is required for interpretation of raw scores for CBS or IBS. Toward this end, height and weight norms were established so that raw CBS and IBS scores could be interpreted in terms of standardized scores. Normal weight, noneating disorder subjects (n = 425) were grouped in terms of CBS, IBS, height, and weight using cluster analysis. A three-cluster solution produced the best separation of CBS and IBS. Cross-validation with a separate sample replicated the three cluster solution. The entire sample was then combined for establishment of norms based upon height and weight of the same subject.

The purpose of the cluster analysis was to establish norms. Means and standard deviations for each cluster were used to establish t scores with a mean of 50 and standard deviation of 10 (norms can be found in Williamson, Davis, et al., in press). Normative data for obese populations have not been established. The norm-referenced data may be used to determine the degree to which a particular individual has a body image disturbance. For example, suppose a female who is 65 in. tall and weighs 125 lbs. chooses the silhouette labeled #7 as her current body size and the silhouette #3 as her ideal body size. Her raw score for current body size (#7) corresponds to a t-score of 70 indicating that she is 2 standard deviations above the norm for females of her height and weight. In other words, this response indicates that this individual perceives herself to be much larger than other females of her same size view themselves. Thus, body image *distortion* is evident. The card chosen for ideal body size (#3) corresponds to a t-score of 37, indicating that this individual is between 1 and 2 standard deviations below the norm for females of her size. In other words, this response is indicative of a stronger *preference for thinness* than other females of the same size. The last piece of information that may be derived from the BIA procedure is the individual's degree of body size dissatisfaction. Note that her current body size is substantially larger than her ideal body size. If her ideal size score (37) is subtracted from her current size score (70), a difference score of (+)33 is obtained. Thus, a high degree of body size *dissatisfaction* is also evident. Note that the difference score of zero (0) would indicate the absence of body size dissatisfaction.

The BIA has been evaluated in terms of reliability and validity. Test-retest estimates have been investigated with the BIA across time intervals ranging from 1 to 8 weeks. Test-retest correlations of .90 for CBS and .71 for IBS were obtained (Williamson, Davis, et al., in press).

Discriminant validity studies have shown the BIA to differentiate bulimia nervosa and normal subjects, in that bulimics chose a larger CBS and thinner IBS than same-sized normals (Williamson et al., 1985). Also, this procedure has been shown to differentiate compulsive overeaters from bulimia nervosa (Davis, Williamson, Goreczny, & Bennett, 1989).

In a study utilizing the BIA, Williamson, Davis, Goreczny, and Blouin (1989) found that bulimia nervosa subjects perceived themselves as larger than same-sized normals across weight levels (from very thin to obese) indicating a body size *distortion* at all weight levels (see Figure 4.3a). Thus, regardless of actual weight level, all bulimia nervosa subjects viewed themselves as larger than nonbulimic subjects of the same weight. As shown in Figure 4.3b, all bulimia nervosa subjects also preferred to be thinner than their same-sized counterparts, indicating a strong *preference for thinness* at all weight levels. Figure 4.3c includes both CBS and IBS scores for bulimia nervosa subjects and nonbulimics. The shaded area signifies the degree of body size dissatisfaction at each weight level for nonbulimics and the horizontal bars signify the degree of body image dissatisfaction for bulimina nervosa subjects, across weight levels. Of particular interest in this study is the finding that all bulimics, except those at extremely low body weight, chose an ideal figure smaller than their current figure, thus indicating body size *dissatisfaction* at virtually all weight levels. Control subjects, in contrast, chose an ideal figure which was larger than their current figure when very thin (i.e., less than 100 lbs). Ideal size

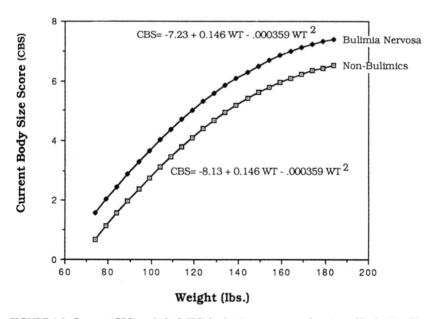

FIGURE 4.3. Current (CBS) and ideal (IBS) body size scores as a function of body size. The upper frame depicts CBS scores for bulimics and controls. The middle frame depicts IBS scores for both groups. The bottom frame combines the data from the other two frames and is published with permission by the American Psychiatric Association [from Williamson, D. A., et al., 1989, p. 98].

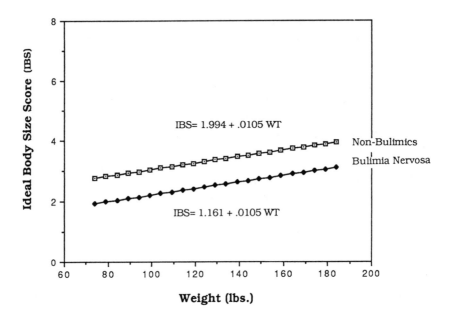

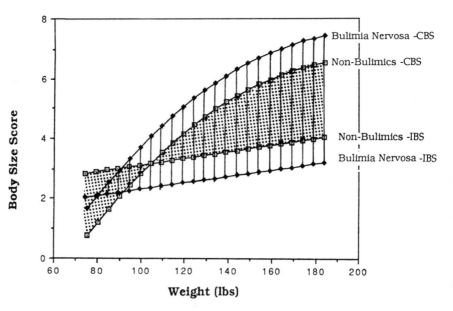

FIGURE 4.3. (*Continued*).

was found to be identical to current size when at a low-normal weight level (i.e., approximately 100 lbs.), and smaller than their current figure when overweight (i.e., greater than 100 lbs.).

These data may help explain some of the conflicting evidence concerning body image disturbances in anorexia and bulimia nervosa. Figure 4.3c shows that as weight decreases the discrepancy between CBS and IBS decreases for the bulimic group and becomes zero at very low weight levels. Anorexics who have achieved a very low weight level often report "satisfaction" with their current size and do not feel "fat," nor do they wish to lose further weight. This clinical description is consistent with the data of Figure 4.3, that is, at very low weight levels bulimics and anorexics may not display body size dissatisfaction. This phenomenon should be studied using other methodology since it may account for the failure to find body image disturbances in anorexics and low weight bulimics.

In conclusion, the BIA has been found to be a reliable, valid, and easily administered procedure. The reliability of this measure has been found to be satisfactory. Also, validity studies have shown the BIA to differentiate bulimia nervosa from normals and compulsive overeaters. The procedure is very easy to use and norms are available to determine the degree to which an individual exhibits body size distortion, preference for thinness, and body size dissatisfaction.

Summary

Current research suggests that body image disturbance can best be understood by analyzing it in terms of its elements. This behavior analytic approach is unique in the history of the study of body image. It is the belief of these authors that this approach will lead to further progress which has eluded traditional psychological researchers and clinicians. A continuation of research designed to investigate body image disturbance in eating disorders is sorely needed so that the construct may become better understood and more clearly defined. Treatment of body image is currently in its infancy. Perhaps development of a better understanding of the specific elements of body image disturbance will lead to improved treatment methods.

Chapter 5
Assessment of Secondary Psychopathology

Earlier chapters have described the assessment of the core psychopathology of eating disorders. This chapter presents procedures for assessing common secondary psychopathology associated with eating disorders. Several studies have reported associations between eating disorders and other problems (e.g., Johnson, Stuckey, Lewis, & Schwartz, 1982, Marcus & Wing, 1987; Prather & Williamson, 1988; Weiss & Ebert, 1983; Williamson, Kelley, Davis, Ruggiero, & Blouin, 1985). Eating disorders have been found to be associated with depression, interpersonal sensitivity, various personality disorders, interpersonal and family problems, anxiety, obsessiveness, substance abuse, and stress. In Figures 1.4, 1.5, and 1.6, bidirectional arrows are used to indicate that we conceptualize these secondary problems to covary with the core symptoms of compulsive overeating, anorexia nervosa, and bulimia nervosa. In other words, these models postulate that secondary problems exacerbate the core eating disorders and vice-versa. While the etiological importance of these secondary psychological problems may be debated, the fact that these problems are frequently seen in eating disorder populations can hardly be questioned. Therefore, from the perspective of properly treating eating disorders, it is imperative that these secondary problems are evaluted and incorporated into a comprehensive treatment plan. We have found that secondary psychopathology often interferes with the treatment process. Therefore direct treatment of problems not directly related to eating may circumvent later difficulties. Some studies (Giles, Young, & Young, 1985; Lacey, 1983; Stevens & Salisbury, 1984) have suggested that nonresponders to eating disorder treatment programs may be those with more severe secondary psychopathology.

This chapter will summarize the primary assessment instruments used for evaluating secondary psychopathology. When possible, "normative" data derived from studies of anorexia nervosa, bulimia nervosa, compulsive overeating, and obesity will be presented. The purpose of presenting these data is to provide the clinician a sense of what to expect when administering a particular instrument to a certain type of patient. From this research, a screening protocol for secondary psychopathology is proposed for use in clinical settings.

SCREENING INSTRUMENTS

The clinician may wish to use a measure of general personality characteristics to screen for secondary psychopathology. Two such instruments that we have found to be most useful are the Minnesota Multiphasic Personality Inventory (MMPI; Hathaway & McKinley, 1951) and the Millon Clinical Multiaxial Inventory (MCMI; Millon, 1982). The MCMI has the advantage of conceptually corresponding more closely to the current diagnostic system than the MMPI, and it is more brief to administer. However, because many items on this instrument load on more than one subscale, the various scales of the MCMI are highly intercorrelated. Because of this psychometric problem, it is not clear whether the MCMI measures different apsects of personality or is primarily a general measure of neuroticism (cf. Choca, Peterson, & Shanley, 1986; Piersma, 1986; Gilbertini & Retzlaff, 1988). Because of these and other problems with the MCMI we recommend using the MMPI as the primary screening instrument for overall psychopathology. Furthermore, a greater number of studies have reported MMPI results for the various eating disorders.

Figure 5.1 illustrates the mean MMPI profiles derived from several studies of eating disorders (Edwin, Andersen, & Rosell, 1988; Prather & Williamson, 1988; Small, Madero, Gross, Teagno, Leib, & Ebert, 1981; Williamson, Kelley, Davis, Ruggiero, & Blouin, 1985). It is readily apparent that all of the eating disorders have similar MMPI profile configurations. The major distinction among the groups is the degree of scale elevations. Note that the general MMPI pattern from group to group suggests that anorexics have the highest scale elevations, followed by bulimics, binge eaters, and obese groups.

Figure 5.1 shows that the most common two-point elevations for all four eating disorder groups on the MMPI are on scales 2 (D) and 4 (Pd). Patients with elevations on scales 2 and 4 have been reported to have poor impulse control. In addition to being impulsive, they often experience a great deal of guilt and anxiety regarding their impulsive behavior. Some reports (e.g., Newark, 1979) have also associated this profile with drug or alcohol abuse and serious family problems.

An MMPI profile which is common to restricting anorexics is elevations

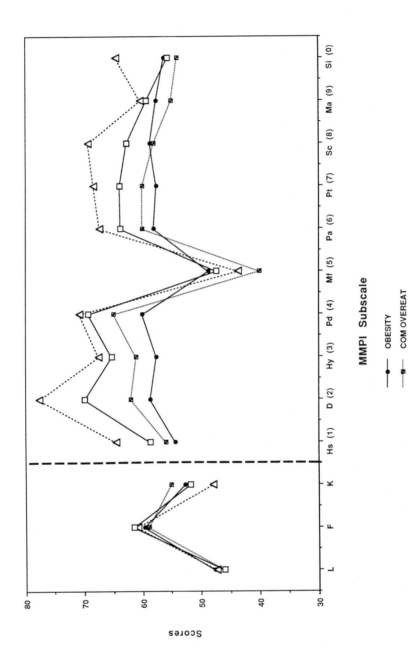

FIGURE 5.1. Mean MMPI profiles for anorexia nervosa, bulimia nervosa, compulsive overeaters, and obesity.

on scales 2 (D), 4 (Pd), 7 (Pt), and 8 (Sc). Patients with elevations on these scales report significant anxiety and depression symptoms. These patients may also feel alienated and may withdraw and avoid close relationships. They also tend to have a history of poor social adjustment. Prognosis of psychological treatment for these patients is reportedly poor, and if scale 8 (Sc) is elevated above 85 the clinician should rule out delusions and/or hallucinations.

Figure 5.1 also suggests that many eating disorder clients have a low scale 5 on the MMPI relative to a high scale 4. Some (e.g., Newark, 1979) have described patients with this configuration to be angry women who are unable to express these feelings directly, leading to a high degree of passive-aggressiveness.

Despite the problems noted earlier, the MCMI can be used to supplement the MMPI. We have used it extensively in recent years and have developed a considerable base of data. The MCMI was designed to assist in diagnosis of axis I and axis II DSM-III disorders. This instrument contains 11 subscales that correspond to DSM personality disorders, 3 of which are called "severe personality disorders." Also, the MCMI has 9 clinical scales which tap various axis I problem areas such as anxiety and depression.

Mean MCMI base rate scores for compulsive overeaters, bulimia nervosa, and anorexia nervosa are summarized in Table 5.1. We did not have an adequate sample of obese patients to provide "normative" data for this measure. Millon (1982) advises that base rate elevations above 84 should be interpreted as the most prominant personality syndromes or clinical symptoms. Elevations above 75 on the MCMI are suggestive of personality or symptom features. Examination of Table 5.1 shows that data from the MCMI corresponds very well to the findings based on the MMPI. Generally, anorexics and bulimics scored higher than compulsive overeaters on most subscales and had a larger number mean scale elevations. Problems of anxiety, dysthymia, and personality disorders were the most common types of secondary psychopathology identified by the MCMI.

DEPRESSION

Clinical studies have consistently found depression to be associated with bulimia, anorexia nervosa, compulsive overeating, and severe cases of obesity (e.g., Marcus & Wing, 1987; Prather & Williamson, 1988; Weiss & Ebert, 1983; Williamson et al., 1985). Lee, Rush, and Mitchell (1985), found that 77 percent of their bulimic sample had at least mild depression. Various symptoms of depression may exacerbate the eating problem (e.g., low activity, appetite changes), and we have found that negative affect often precedes binging.

Table 5.1. MCMI Mean Base Rate Scores by
Clinical Group

Subscale	Group		
	CO	AN	BN
Personality Scales			
Schizoid	57	54	65
Avoidant	64	66	78*
Dependent	79*	65	87**
Histrionic	60	55	44
Narcissistic	57	53	39
Antisocial	41	55	37
Compulsive	54	56	48
Passive/Aggressive	62	73	76*
Schizotypal	63	59	64
Borderline	67	76*	75*
Paranoid	54	56	51
Clinical Scales			
Anxiety	76*	87**	92**
Somatoform	62	70	76*
Hypomania	51	51	45
Dysthmia	71	85**	84*
Alcohol Abuse	56	61	58
Drug Abuse	49	52	47
Psychotic Thinking	58	60	63
Psychotic Depression	61	64	67
Psychotic Delusions	53	56	56

CO = Compulsive Overeaters, AN = Anorexia Nervosa, BN = Bulimia Nervosa

Single asterisks signify mean scale elevations above the cutoff score for symptom features, i.e., 70. Double asterisks indicate mean base rate scores above the clinical cutoff of 84.

Depression is so common to bulimia that some have suggested that it is simply an "affective variant" (Pope & Hudson, 1985). This theory proposes that the core underlying psychopathology of bulimia is major depression. While this is a tempting notion because of the known appetite disturbances the affective disorders cause, several reviews (e.g., Hinz & Williamson, 1987; Wilson & Lindholm, 1987) have concluded that the evidence for depression as the *cause* of bulimia is not convincing, and that bulimia is best conceptualized as being associated with secondary depression, much as depression is a common secondary problem associated with obsessive-compulsive disorder.

Several structured interviews have been developed for assessing depression. Two of the most frequently used clinician rating scales are the Schedule for Affective Disorders and Schizophrenia (SADS; Endicott &

Spitzer, 1978) and the Hamilton Rating Scale for Depression (HRSD; Hamilton, 1960; 1967). The SADS was developed from the Research Diagnostic Criteria (Spitzer, Endicott, & Robins, 1975; 1978) and was intended to provide structured information following standardized operational criteria. Thus, this measure covers the symptoms of depression comprehensively, and is a psychometrically sound instrument for the diagnosis of affective disorders.

The HRSD is an interview scale that should be used primarily for assessing the severity of depression. Outpatient means for the 17-item version of this scale vary from 24 to 27, while inpatients tend to score more in the range of 30 to 44. Lee et al. (1985) found that 53 percent of their bulimic population scored over 18 on the 24-item version of this measure. This instrument may be valuable to assess treatment gains as it appears to be sensitive to clinical change.

Because the clinician may not wish to take the necessary time to administer measures like the SADS or the HRSD, Appendix C contains a relatively brief interview that may be used to help in assessing the level of depression. We have called this instrument the Brief Interview of Secondary Psychopathology (BISP). This interview contains 9 basic question areas relating to both depression and anxiety. These questions yield client responses which aid the clinician's rating of 15 symptom areas relating to depression and anxiety. Thus, this relatively brief interview gives the clinician direction as to what mood or anxiety disorders the eating disorder client may be experiencing, as well as giving the evaluator a simple determination of the patient's level of depression or anxiety. This interview may be used in assessing a client's progress in these areas as well. Following the anxiety/depression section, this interview contains questions related to social relationships and substance use.

Numerous self-report scales exist for assessing depression. We find the Beck Depression Inventory (BDI; Beck & Beamesderfer, 1974) to be quite useful. This measure is simple to administer, short, and easy to score. Suggested cutoffs are 0–10, normal mood fluctuations; 11–18, subclinical mood disturbance; 18–30, mild to moderate depression; 30–40, severe depression; and greater than 40 as indicative of extreme depression. Beck and Beamesderfer (1974) also suggest that any patient scoring above 13 on the BDI should be investigated further to rule out depression. Table 5.2 lists mean scores from several studies of various self-report depression measures, including the BDI. As this table demonstrates, anorexics tend to score the highest on the BDI, followed by bulimics, and compulsive overeaters, with BDI scores for obese subjects being quite lower than the other eating disorders groups. Various studies report mean BDI scores of bulimic patients ranging from 15 to 22, with high frequency purgers tending to score in the upper end of this range (Williamson, Prather, Upton,

Table 5.2. Mean Scores of Depression Measures by Clinical Group

Assessment Instruments	Purpose	Mean Scores				References
		Ob	CO	AN	BN	
BDI	Assess level of depression	10	17	19	18	Marcus & Wing, 1987
CES-D	Assess depressive symptoms	21	30	30	27	Prather, 1989
SCL-90-D (t-scores)	Assess level of depression	61	65	70	67	Prather & Williamson, 1988
PES	Assess					Hood et al., 1982
P	pleasantness (P),	0.78	1.07	0.83	1.10	
F	and frequency of activity (F)	.61	.63	.65	.79	
DAS	Assess dysfunctional attitudes	134	141	136	156	

CO = Compulsive Overeaters, AN = Anorexia Nervosa, BN = Bilimia Nervosa

Davis, Ruggiero, & Van Buren, 1987). Prather and Williamson (1988) found that obese subjects may differ significantly in depression as measured by the BDI, depending on whether they are seeking weight loss treatment. Clients seeking psychological treatment for obesity tend to score higher on this measure.

Other brief self-report scales for depression are the Center for Epidemiological Studies Depression Scale (CES-D; Radloff, 1977) and the depression subscale of the Symptom Checklist-90 (SCL-90-D; Derogatis, 1977). Means for eating disorder subjects on the CES-D and the SCL-90-D are included in Table 5.2. As with the BDI, means of several studies of these measures show that depression is most common in anorexics, and obese patients tend to show less depression than the other eating disorder groups.

If depression is found to be present, the clinician may wish to evaluate characteristics that may be maintaining the depression. Frequently, low activity level or withdrawal from pleasurable activities is associated with depression. Following the approach of Peter Lewinsohn and associates, the Pleasant Events Schedule (PES; MacPhillamy & Lewinsohn, 1974; 1976) was developed to measure the activity level and amount of enjoyment subjects were experiencing in relation to various events. This schedule yields three different scores: a frequency score which is reflective of how much the client engages in these activities, a "pleasantness" score which reveals how much the subject may potentially enjoy these events, and a score which indicates the obtained reinforcement each subject has experienced in the past month. Data gained from the PES in our clinic show that obese subjects report the lowest frequency of activity (approximately one standard deviation below normal subjects), and anorexics score lowest on the pleasantness scale (one standard deviation below the mean). The following example illustrates how the PES is used.

Case Example. Helen was a 42-year-old married woman who had come to seek treatment for weight loss. Throughout the interview, it was clear that she was an obese compulsive overeater. Her BDI score of 22 suggested that she was also moderately depressed. After determining that Helen met the DSM-III-R diagnostic criteria for dysthymia, she was administered the PES. Her frequency score of .59 was over one standard deviation below the mean for her age group. Also her obtained reinforcement score (.90) was about one standard deviation below her age group average. However, Helen's pleasantness score (1.21) was above the mean. This pattern of data suggested that Helen had the potential for experiencing pleasure associated with various activities, but that she was not engaging in these activities on a regular basis. Therefore, her treatment plan targeted increased activity with the expectation that it should help her lose weight and should be maintained by naturally occurring reinforcers.

Negativistic thinking has also been strongly associated with depression. One self-report instrument which we have found to be a useful measure of negativistic thinking is the Dysfunctional Attitudes Scale (DAS; Weissman & Beck, 1978). Nondepressed subjects have been found to score from 105–119 on this scale, while depressed subjects' scores average about 147 (e.g., Hamilton & Abramson, 1983). Although the total DAS score may alert the clinician to the presence of dysfunctional attitudes, the global score does not specify the specific content of negativistic thinking. Thus, we find that individual item analysis of this measure is useful in determining what dysfunctional attitudes may be targeted in treatment. Means of eating disorders subjects for both the PES and the DAS are found in Table 5.2. The DAS means for all four eating disorder groups are more than one standard deviation above the mean for normals, with bulimics reporting the most severe negativistic thinking.

ANXIETY

As noted earlier, anxiety is also frequently associated with eating disorders. Anxiety seems to be associated more frequently with bulimia and anorexia nervosa and is most obviously related to fear of weight gain. We have found that eating disorder patients also experience considerable anxiety about other problems as well. The clinical interview is an important tool for assessing problems related to anxiety. One of the best structured interviews for anxiety is the Anxiety Disorder Interview Schedule (ADIS; DiNardo, O'Brien, Barlow, Waddell, & Blanchard, 1983). The ADIS includes the Hamilton Rating Scale for Anxiety (HRSA; Hamilton, 1959), and was developed for differential diagnosis of the anxiety disorders specified by DSM-III. Unfortunately, the ADIS is a very lengthy interview format, often requiring more than two hours to administer. The structured interview in Appendix C is fairly brief in administration and provides the evaluator with information regarding anxiety symptoms and level of severity. We recommend that if a patient scores greater than 6 on anxiety symptoms, then more intensive evaluation of anxiety problems should be conducted to rule out a specific anxiety disorder.

Several self-report instruments have been developed for assessing anxiety problems. Data related to these questionnaires are summarized in Table 5.3. The State-Trait Anxiety Inventory (STAI; Speilberger, Gorsuch, & Lushene, 1970) can be used for evaulating current (state) anxiety as well as the extent of anxiety a subject generally experiences (trait anxiety). Data from our clinic (see Table 5.3) show that none of the groups averaged state or trait scores more than two standard deviations above the mean (i.e., t-scores greater than 70). Obese subjects were found to score at about the mean of 50 and anorexia nervosa, bulimia nervosa, and compulsive overeaters scored within one and one-half standard deviations above the mean.

The anxiety subscale of the MCMI or the anxiety subscale of the SCL-90 (SCL-90-A; Derogatis, 1977) can also be used as an index of generalized anxiety. Elevations on scales 7 (Pt) and 8 (Sc) of the MMPI also sug-

Table 5.3. Mean Scores of Anxiety Measures by Clinical Group

Assessment Instrument	Purpose	Mean Scores				References
		Ob	CO	AN	BN	
STAI-State (t-scores)	Assess current anxiety level	41	56	60	53	Prather, 1989
STAI-Trait (t-scores)	Assess general anxiety level	49	65	58	58	
SCL-90-Anx (t-scores)	Assess general anxiety symptoms	57	62	68	65	Prather & Williamson, 1988

CO = Compulsive Overeaters, AN = Anorexia Nervosa, BN = Bulimia Nervosa

gest a significant level of anxiety and worry. As shown in Tables 5.1 and 5.3, anorexics and bulimics tend to score higher on these measures of anxiety with simple obesity patients reporting the least anxiety.

OBSESSIVE-COMPULSIVE HABITS

While estimates vary, obsessive-compulsive features are apparently fairly common in anorexics (Dally, 1969; Halmi, 1974; Theander, 1970). Kasvikis, Tsakiris, Marks, Basoglu, and Noshirvani (1986) found that 16 of 151 female obsessive-compulsives had a past history of anorexia nervosa. Also, Hudson, Pope, Yurgelin-Todd, Jonas, and Frankenburg (1987) reported that 33% of their bulimic population (n = 51) could be classified as meeting the diagnostic criteria for obsessive-compulsive disorder at some time in their lives.

We have found that Maudsley Obsessional-Compulsive Inventory (MOCI; Hodgson & Rachman, 1977) to be a useful self-report inventory for measuring obsessive-compulsive symptoms of checking rituals, washing rituals, slowness, and doubting-conscientiousness. Also, the obsessive-compulsive subscale of the SCL-90 may be used as a general measure of obsessiveness (SCL-90-OC; Derogatis, 1977). Table 5.4 contains mean scores for eating disorder subjects on these measures. These data suggest that anorexics tend to have the worst problems with obsessive-compulsiveness. In particular, the mean for anorexics on the slowness factor of the MOCI is approximately one standard deviation above the mean Hodgson and Rachman (1977) reported for neurotics and is close to the average score reported for obsessionals in this study.

Table 5.4. Mean Scores of Obsessive-Compulsive Habits Measures

Assessment Instrument	Purpose	Mean Scores				References
		Ob	CO	AN	BN	
SCL-90-OC	Assess level of obsessive compulsive symptoms	58	63	72	64	Prather & Williamson, 1988
MOCI	Assess					
-checking	obsessive	#	2.2	3.4	2.5	
-washing	habits, with	#	2.2	3.4	2.4	
-slowness	four scales	#	1.9	3.4	2.4	
-doubting		#	4.0	4.5	3.6	

CO = Compulsive Overeaters, AN = Anorexia Nervosa, BN = Bulimia Nervosa

INTERPERSONAL SENSITIVITY

Social anxiety is especially problematic for many eating disorder patients. Obese persons may not want to be seen in public, and bulimics or anorexics may be overly concerned about how others are evaluating their appearance or their eating habits. Interpersonal sensitivity may be defined as overconcern regarding the behaviors and opinions of others that a person perceives are directed toward him or her. If a compulsive eater consistently avoids social interactions then he or she will probably spend more time at home, which frequently is an environment in which the client is vulnerable to overeating. In addition, feelings of rejection or negative evauality may lead to binging epidoses with many eating disorder patients.

It is very important to determine whether a patient's interpersonal problems are due to social anxiety, poor interpersonal skills, or both. Many patients are very sensitive to social feedback and frequently misinterpret the statements or actions of others in a negativistic manner. The "interpersonal sensitivity" subscale of the SCL-90 (SCL-90-IS; Derogatis, 1977) and/or the Fear of Negative Evaluation scale (FNE; Watson & Friend, 1969) may be used for assessing this type of social anxiety. Table 5.5 lists mean scores for eating disorder patients on these measures. These data suggest that anorexics have the greatest degree of interpersonal sensitivity. Bulimics and compulsive overeaters also were found to have significant anxiety related to interpersonal situations.

The social introversion subscale on the MMPI (MMPI-Si) may also provide useful data regarding interpersonal problems of eating disorder patients. This scale is a stable measure of an individual's social activity and how comfortable a person is in interpersonal relations. Moderate elevations on this scale are typical of reserved individuals who are somewhat shy. Individuals with high MMPI-Si elevations (>70) are usually very aware of their social discomfort. These individuals may also be seen as

Table 5.5. Mean Scores by Group Relating to Interpersonal Sensitivity

Assessment Instrument	Purpose	Mean Scores				References
		Ob	CO	AN	BN	
SCL-90-IS	Assess symptoms of interpersonal sensitivity	62	68	73	68	Prather & Williamson, 1988
FNE	Measures fear of negative evaluation	24	21	25	18	

CO = Compulsive Overeaters, AN = Anorexia Nervosa, BN = Bulimia Nervosa

introverted, in addition to lacking self-confidence. Referring back to Figure 5.1 shows that the response of eating disorder subjects on this scale is parallel to those on the SCL-90-IS and the FNE in that anorexics scored higher on MMPI-Si (0) than the other eating disorder groups.

INTERPERSONAL AND FAMILY PROBLEMS

Individuals with an eating disorder are often overly dependent on one or a very few relationships. For example, with some patients all social activity may evolve around one particular friend or family member. This individual is frequently the patient's spouse or romantic partner. This dependency often causes considerable stress for the partner, and if the relationship fails, quite often the patient's social world falls apart. It is easy to understand how those who have a high degree of interpersonal sensitivity may be overly dependent on a few relationships. If forming interpersonal relationships produces emotional discomfort, it follows that such an individual would try to form a very few, intense relationships. Thus, dependent personality features are a very important interpersonal problem to evaluate. This topic is discussed in more detail in the subsequent section dealing with personality disorders.

In addition to social anxiety, eating disorder clients may have frequent conflict with significant others. At times this conflict appears to be due to oversensitivity on the part of the patient, and other times it may be due to an insensitivity on the part of those who are close to the patient. One section of the BISP (Appendix C) asks questions about the frequency and types of interpersonal conflict experienced by the patient. If frequent conflict is found to occur, then the interview should investigate when and with whom conflicts typically occur, and the "topics" or situations which lead to conflict. Also the consequences (aftereffects) of interpersonal conflict should be thoroughly investigated since negative affect often increases the likelihood of problematic eating behavior. For example, a bulimic college student may have a heated argument with her boyfriend leading to her "storming" back to the dorm. Once in her dorm room, she may binge and purge in a "fit" of anger. Following this emotional outburst, the patient's boyfriend may call her, apologize for the conflict, and offer some recompense for his actions. In a situation such as this, the clinician should note not only the tendency to engage in the problem behavior of eating following the conflict, but also how her boyfriend's response to the conflict may reinforce maladaptive conflict resolution and the use of bulimic habits for the purpose of stress management.

A common area of interpersonal conflict is with family members, in particular with parents and siblings, or with spouse and children.

While the earliest accounts of anorexia emphasized family variables as important in the development of this disorder (e.g., Bruch, 1973; Minuchin, Rosman, & Baker, 1978), currently it is unclear as to exactly how family factors may be involved with etiology (cf. Strober & Humphrey, 1987). Our experience suggests that family problems are frequent enough to make family therapy a critical aspect of treatment for most of our patients. In addition to being implicated in the development of eating disorders, family problems may also be caused by the disorder itself. For example, the secretive behavior of the bulimic or the defiant behavior of the anorexic patient may cause considerable conflict and loss of trust among family members. The following case example illustrates how a patient's eating disorder problems may contribute to conflict and misunderstanding among family members.

Case Example. Ashley was a college sophomore, living at home with her family. She had two brothers and her family was very close. Her father was a civil engineer working at a local power company. Ashley had been referred to the eating disorders clinic by the family dentist, who suspected bulimia after a routine dental examination. Initial assessment found that Ashley met the diagnostic criteria for bulimia nervosa. Although Ashley had always been quite close to her parents, in the past year their relationship had deteriorated and neither Ashley nor her parents were sure why this deterioration had occurred. Upon interviewing her parents, it was discovered that the family dinner was a very important family activity. Recently, Ashley had refused to eat with the family, and when she did eat with them, her parents noticed that she ate very little, if any, of her food. Not only had this behavior produced family conflict, but Ashley's mother complained that she was spending more and more time alone in her room and "away from the family." Ashley had claimed that this isolation was required by the demands of studying, but further investigation found that she frequently binged and purged while alone in her room. Ashley had increased her isolation as binging and purging had increased in frequency. Since the family was unaware of her bulimic habits, they attributed her isolation and failure to eat with the family as indicative of rejection by Ashley. These issues were addressed in the first few sessions of family therapy.

The clinician should also evaluate the psychosocial characteristics of the family. Research from our clinic (Head, Williamson, Duchman, & Bennett, 1988) has suggested that the families of bulimics are characteristically low in cohesion and seldom freely allow expression of emotion. Conflict among family members is also quite common. These findings are consistent with other published studies of the families of anorexics and bulimics. It should be noted, however, that similar family backgrounds have also been found with psychiatric problems other than eating disorders (cf. Strober & Humphrey, 1987). Head et al. (1988) found that family problems were more strongly associated with secondary psychopathology than to problems related to eating. Thus, it is important to assess for significant family problems, but one should not assume that because a person has an eating disorder that family problems must be found. While family disruptions are frequent, often quite normal family environments are found, especially when the patient has only recently developed an eating disorder.

Several self-report measures have been developed for the evaluation of family problems. The Family Environment Scale (FES; Moos & Moos, 1980, 1986) is useful for providing a general profile of a person's family characteristics. This instrument has ten factors: cohesion, expressiveness, conflict, independence, achievement orientation, intellectual/cultural orientation, active/recreational orientation, moral/religious emphasis, organization, and control. Table 5.6 summarizes the results on the FES for the various eating disorder groups. These data suggest that the families of anorexics and bulimics characteristically are low in cohesiveness, expression of emotion, and experience a great deal of conflict. The families of compulsive overeater groups did not encourage independence of the family members.

Marital conflict may also detract from treatment. Van Buren and Williamson (1988) found that married bulimic patients were very similar to those seeking marital therapy. They were generally dissatisfied with their

Table 5.6. Mean Scores of Instruments Relating to Interpersonal and Family Problems

Assessment Instrument	Purpose	Mean Scores				References
		Ob	CE	AN	BN	
FES (t-scores)	General assessment family characteristics					Ordman & Kirschenbaum, 1986
Cohesion		34	42	34	28	Head et al. 1988
Expression		41	41	37	35	
Conflict		51	54	59	59	
Independence		32	32	36	38	
Achievement		44	50	50	54	
Intellectual		32	41	41	39	
Recreational		35	43	43	45	
Religious		51	51	54	50	
Organization		42	48	53	49	
Control		56	56	56	56	
DAS	Measures marital adjustment				86 (98)	Van Buren & Williamson, 1988

Ob = Obese, CO = Compulsive Overeaters, AN = Anorexia Nervosa, BN = Bulimia Nervosa marital relationship, used passive problem-solving skills, withdrew from conflict, and expressed the belief that their partners could not change. Thus, marital difficulties may be a common problem for older eating disorder patients. If, through interview, the clinician determines that this is an area that may need attention in treatment, several self-report measures may be useful. The Dyadic Adjustment Scale (DAS; Spanier, 1976) and the Marital Satisfaction Inventory (MSI; Snyder, 1979) are two of the most popular instruments that assess marital satisfaction.

PERSONALITY DISORDERS

In our clinic, about 35 percent of eating disorder cases also receive pesonality disorder diagnoses. In utilizing the MCMI, Head et al. (1988) found that the most common personality disorders in bulimics were dependent, avoidant, passive-aggressive, and borderline personality disorders. Piran, Lerner, Garfinkel, Kennedy, and Brouillete (1988) reported that bulimics tended to receive personality diagnoses of borderline (39.5%) and histrionic (13.1%), while anorexics were frequently diagnosed as avoidant (33%) and dependent (10%) personality disorders.

The diagnosis of personality disorders is important because these personality variables often interfere with treatment. It is common to see patients who receive secondary gain by engaging in anorexic or bulimic eating patterns. For example, the passive-aggressive personality disorder may receive considerable negative attention from her or his family for dysfunctional eating behavior which serves to maintain the problematic eating habits. Borderline patients may be quite compliant with treatment one day, but sabotage the treatment program the next day. Recognition of these personality characteristics and their interaction with problems of eating are essential if treatment is to be conducted without serious pitfalls.

Few measures have been developed to assess the presence of personality disorders directly. We have found the MCMI (Millon, 1982) to serve as a useful screening instrument for personality disorders. Table 5.1 summarizes MCMI mean base rate scores for the four eating disorder groups. These data show that dependent personality features are quite common in bulimia nervosa and to a lesser degree in compulsive overeaters. Avoidant and passive-aggressive traits were also commonly observed in bulimia nervosa. Of the more severe personality disorders, borderline personality characteristics are frequently associated with anorexia and bulimia. We find that the subscale scores of the MCMI cannot be used for personality disorder diagnoses. Instead, results from the MCMI should help to direct interview queries to formally rule out a personality disturbance.

The clinician may also use the MMPI as a screening instrument for personality disorders. Borderline patients typically exhibit 4-6-2 or 4-8-2 configurations on the MMPI. Individuals with dependent personality often have elevations on scales 2 (D) and 7 (Pt). MMPI elevations on scale 2 (D) and scale 0 (Si) may indicate an avoidant or schizoid personality. Passive-aggressive individuals, on the other hand, may have elevations on scales 3 (Hy) and 4 (Pd). As noted earlier, an elevated scale 4 (Pd) in combination with a low scale 5 (Mf) may also suggest a passive-aggressive personality. Two point elevations on scales 3 (Hy) and 1 (Hs) are associated with histrionic features, particularly when scale 3 is significantly above scale 1.

The FNE and the SCL-90-Interpersonal Sensitivity subscale can also be used for detecting avoidant personality disorder. Fear of negative evaluation and interpersonal sensitivity are important components of this personality disturbance, and thus these measures can be beneficial for this evaluation. Also, we have found high scores on the FNE in dependent patients as well.

SUBSTANCE ABUSE

Studies vary as to what proportion of eating disorder patients have additional problems with substance abuse. Most studies have found that substance abuse is more prevalent in the eating disorders than in the general population (e.g., Bulik, 1987). A recent study (Hudson, Weiss, Pope, McElroy, & Mirin, in press) found that 15% of 143 women hospitalized for substance abuse could have been diagnosed as bulimic or anorexic at some point in their life. These patients often abused stimulants in order to suppress appetite. Alcohol is also frequently abused by bulimics and compulsive overeaters. Hood, Moore, and Garner (1982) found that cigarette use was even more common than alcohol use in their anorexic population (47% vs. 15%). Unpublished data from our clinic confirm this finding with bulimics. These data show that bulimics tend to give dietary reasons for avoiding alcohol and for smoking cigarettes, suggesting that fear of weight gain may contribute to substance use in anorexia and bulimia.

Problems with alcohol or other drugs can impair treatment. We have found that some bulimics will be much more likely to binge and purge after a few drinks. Thus, the clinician should not overlook the possibility for problems in this area. Two structured interviews may be useful for obtaining information related to alcohol abuse. The Drinking Profile (Marlatt, 1976) is a commonly used interview procedure. This interview takes about one hour to administer. The Time-Line technique (Sobell, Maisto, Sobell, & Cooper 1979) assesses daily drinking for the 360 days prior to the interview. This interview takes approximately 20 to 40 minutes to administer. While clinical lore suggests that we should mistrust the reports of those being treated for substance abuse, several recent reviews have cast doubt on this assumption (e.g., Sobell & Sobell, 1986). It is true that self-report is unreliable with a small proportion of substance abusers. It appears, however, that most can be trusted to report their substance use fairly accurately.

Two of the most commonly used self-report instruments for substance abuse are the Michigan Alcoholism Screening Test (MAST; Selzer, 1971) and the Drug Abuse Screening Test (DAST; Skinner, 1982). Both take only about 5 minutes to complete. If the clinician suspects problems with substance abuse, several objective techniques may be used. But the clinician should be warned not to rely heavily on these techniques as they also have shortcomings (cf. Salaspuro, 1986). For alcohol use the breath alcohol tests are convenient and give the clinician immediate feedback as to alcohol use. There now exist several inexpensive portable breath analyzers (cf. Sobell & Sobell, 1975). A new technique is the alcohol dipstick (Kapur & Israel, 1983). The dipstick is placed into the urine, saliva, or blood, and results in different color intensities which relate to different ethanol levels. If one wishes to get an objective assessment of multiple drug use, urinalysis is advised. Although this technique is relatively expensive and results are not immediate, it can provide quite accurate assessment of the type of drug use, and in some cases the amount of drug found in the body.

STRESS

Assessment of environmental stressors may be important for understanding the onset of an eating disorder and in determining maintenance factors. Commonly cited events preceding the onset of eating disorders include change of home, change of school or college, serious illness of family member, and separation from a friend (Gomez & Dally, 1980; Pyle, Mitchell, & Eckert, 1981). Common stressors such as family arguments are frequently reported by eating disorder patients. Recent research (Kanner, Coyne, Schaefer, & Lazarus, 1981; Delongis, Coyne, Dakof, Folkman, & Lazarus, 1982) has shown that these "minor" stressors are more predictive of psychological and somatic symptoms than are major stressors. Further, these authors also point out that daily stressors are much more amenable to psychological treatment than are major life stressors. Thus, it may be more important to assess these daily stressors or "hassles" than major life events such as marriage, divorce, loss of job, death of relative, and so forth.

Two measures have been developed for this purpose: the Hassles Scale (Kanner et al., 1981) and the Daily Stress Inventory (DSI; Brantley, Waggoner, Jones, & Rappaport, 1987). The Hassles scale was designed to measure the frequency and impact of hassles in the last month. Kanner et al. (1981, p. 3) define hassles as "the irritating, frustrating, distressing demands that to some degree characterize everyday transactions with the environment." Subjects rate 117 common hassles on this scale for the past month. This instrument yields two scores: frequency, which is the total number of items checked, and intensity, which is the mean severity per item rated by the subject. Content areas for the hassles are work, family, social activities, environment, practical considerations (such as misplacing things), finances, and health. Thus, with the administration of this scale, the clinician can identify life problems that may lead to problem eating episodes.

The Daily Stress Inventory (DSI) was designed to measure the number of minor stressors and their psychological impact on a given day (Brantley, Cocke, Jones, & Goreczny, 1988). The DSI, unlike the Hassles scale, is used as a daily self-monitoring instrument. Thus, the DSI has the potential for a more fine-grained analysis of the relationship between stress and eating behavior.

Summary

This chapter reviewed various assessment procedures and research findings related to common secondary psychopathology found in the eating disorders. In reviewing these data, the pattern is quite striking. Across a diversity of measures and problem areas, anorexics generally were found to have the highest levels of secondary psychopathology, followed by bulimics, who are followed by the compulsive overeater and obese groups. This pattern is supportive of the contention made by Williamson, Kelley, Cavell, and Prather (1987) that the secondary problems of eating disorders are like a continuum with anorexia nervosa patients generally expressing the greatest degree of psychopathology and obese patients the least. We hope the data presented in this chapter will serve as a set of "norms" for the four eating disorder groups so that clinicians can judge whether a particular anorexic or bulimic is typical versus more or less severe than the "norm." It is unlikely that the average clinician would elect to use all of the instruments and procedures presented here. For this reason, we would like to suggest a select set of screening instruments for assessing the secondary psychopathology of eating disorders. These instruments are summarized in Table 5.7. The brief interview given in Appendix C should serve as an adequate interview format. This interview covers the areas of depression, anxiety, obsessive-compulsive habits, interpersonal problems, and substance abuse. The MMPI may be used as a general screening instrument for personality disorders and other clinical

Table 5.7. Suggested Assessment Protocol for Secondary Psychopathology

Assessment Instrument	Problem Areas	Comments
Brief Interview of Secondary Psychopathology (BISP)	Depression, anxiety, O-C, interpersonal problems, substance abuse	found in appendix
MMPI	General screening, personality problems	
BDI	Depression	
PES	Depression, activity level, reinforcement	use if depressed
DAS	Depression, dysfunctional attitudes	use if depressed
STAI	Anxiety	
MOCI	O-C habits	
FES	Family problems	
DAS	Marital problems	use if marital distress reported
FNE	Interpersonal sensitivity, personality	

problems. The BDI provides an adequate measure for assessing the symptoms and severity of depression. If information from the interview and the BDI suggest that depression might be present, then the clinician may choose to administer the PES and the Dysfunctional Attitudes Scale in order to gather further information about the cognitive versus behavioral factors maintaining the depression. The STAI is also fairly brief, and the information obtained from this self-report inventory, combined with information from the MMPI, should give the clinician sufficient information to rule out anxiety problems. The MOCI can provide additional information about obsessive-compulsive features. The FES can be used to screen for significant family problems, and if the interview indicates possible marital discord, the clinician may wish to administer the Dyadic Adjustment Scale. Finally, the FNE can provide information regarding interpersonal sensitivity and similar problems related to social anxiety. This assessment protocol should require about two hours for most patients and will provide enough information related to secondary psychopathology to allow for proper treatment planning. If further assessment is required, it can be collected at a later date.

Chapter 6
Special Problems
of Assessment

The preceding chapters have discussed methods for conceptualization, assessment, and diagnosis of eating disorders. These procedures are quite useful and straightforward when evaluating a compliant person who recognizes that he or she has an eating disorder, and is volunteering for treatment. But what happens when the patient is not compliant and is being evaluated under coercion by a concerned family? The problem of evaluating the resistant patient occurs frequently when assessing eating disorder patients. Such patients often require inpatient treatment. Assessment of inpatients presents unique problems, but also allows for a more objective evaluation of eating behaviors, weight changes, and so forth. The following sections describe how we have learned to handle these special problems. The first section discusses strategies for evaluating resistant patients. The last section describes some of the assessment options which are unique to evaluation in an inpatient setting.

ASSESSMENT OF THE RESISTANT
PATIENT

Common Problems

Evaluation of the resistant patient presents challenges quite different from those posed by compliant patients who are voluntarily seeking treatment. The resistant patient is usually referred for evaluation by the parents, guardians, or family members seeking some explanation of the person's unusual eating habits. Such cases are most often adolescents, and are usually anorexic or bulimic. Many older anorexics and bulimics can also be quite resistant to the evaluation and treatment process, however.

Due to the initial (and sometimes continuing) resistance, the patient may often attempt to deceive the person(s) conducting the evaluation. This resistance may be manifested in a variety of ways. During assessment, the patient may often minimize or negate any report of affective distress regarding weight gain, eating "normally," or binge eating. School problems (e.g., grades, social interactions, conduct), family problems, or the presence of secondary psychopathology may be similarly minimized. If self-monitoring is a component of the assessment process, the records may be repeatedly "lost" or "forgotten." With paper-and-pencil assessment, the results may show a guarded, or "fake good" pattern of responding. The following case example illustrates some of the problems of assessing the resistant patient.

Case Example. Linda was a 16-year-old female, 5 ft. 6 in. tall and weighing 109 lbs. She was admitted to the hospital by her parents. She had lost 20 lbs. during the previous two months "just to firm up—for health reasons." Her description of recent eating habits suggested that she was eating approximately 1800 calories per day. She was not purging via vomiting, laxatives, diuretics, excessive exercise, appetite suppressants, or restrictive eating. Her results on the MMPI yielded an invalid profile, with an F minus K index of −18. This pattern of test scores strongly suggested that Linda was minimizing the nature of her problems. All clinical scales were below t-scores of 70. On the Beck Depression Inventory, Linda's total score was 3, or within the normal range. On the Eating Attitudes Test, Bulimia Test, Eating Questionnaire-Revised, and Eating Disorder Inventory, Linda's scores were all within the normal range.

Interviews with her mother and father provided a quite different picture. The parents described a pattern of restrictive eating (e.g., no breakfast, small portions of food at dinner) at home, and reports from peers at school indicated that Linda ate very little, if anything, at lunch. Also, Linda's mother had found laxatives in her daughter's bathroom.

When presented with the report of her parents and friends, Linda initially became very angry and tearful, accusing them of lying about her eating. However, with further questioning, she did admit that perhaps she had minimized her problems of eating, and stated that she "occasionally" used laxatives. However, she still refused to offer a complete description of her eating and purgative habits. Based upon the strong evidence of an eating disorder and Linda's continued denial and resistance, a recommendation of inpatient evaluation and treatment was made. Only in a very controlled environment could we expect to evaluate accurately her problems related to eating.

Due to the minimization of symptomatology by resistant patients, reliance upon the report of significant others (e.g., family members, teachers, peers) is an integral facet of the assessment process. Parents, siblings, teachers, and peers can often provide a reasonably accurate report of the patient's eating patterns at home, school, and in social settings. In particular, restrictive eating can be easily noted by others. A common report from family members of an anorexic is one in which the patient makes excuses for not eating, stating that she or he has just eaten (of course, without anyone witnessing the meal), or plans to eat later. These "omissions of eating," however, may often not be noticed by significant others, and therefore the clinician should be careful to ask very direct questions about eating habits and associated problems. For example, asking "Do you get nervous or anxious after you eat?" to an anorexic who is eating only rice cakes and lettuce may elicit an emphatic answer of "No." These foods are considered "safe," and do not cause any degree of emotional discomfort. However, asking "If I asked you to eat a candy bar right now, how would you feel?" may elicit a more accurate description of the emotional consequences of eating forbidden foods.

Compulsive binging and purging are typically very secretive behaviors. The recurrent unexplained disappearance of large amounts of food may be noticed by family members, suggesting the occurrence of binging. Also, family members may note an unusual number of empty food bags and containers in the patient's bathroom or bedroom garbage container, and when properly questioned, may provide data suggestive of frequent binge eating. Evidence of purgative behavior (empty laxative boxes, vomitus in the toilet bowl or sink) may also be noted for a patient who purges. Asking the family about the patient's behavior after eating may also provide information about the possibility of purging. For example, if the patient typically leaves the table immediately after a meal to go to a bathroom, purging may be suspected.

Teachers and peers may be able to provide valuable information about the patient's behavior during meals eaten while in school. Often, the family is unaware of the patient's eating behavior at school, as the patient may not be truthful about eating when away from the scrutiny of the family. Also, information about problems other than eating may be assessed via an interview with teachers. Conduct problems, isolation from peers, decline in school performance, and fatigue may be easily noted by those who have worked with the patient in his or her school setting. Questions about affect, irritability, and peer relationships should also be asked when interviewing significant others.

When the resistant patient begins treatment and is asked to begin eating under the observation of professionals, a more accurate description of the patient's eating style can usually be obtained. Fear of eating and weight gain may be expressed through making "low calorie" food choices, eating only small portions of the meals, and refusing to choose and eat certain "forbidden" foods. Hiding or disposing of foods which are feared is also common. Also, the patient may make consistent and multiple requests to go to the bathroom after eating a meal, or attempt to "slip away" to the bathroom, in hopes of being able to purge. When the patient who reported few problems of eating (but in reality is anorexic or bulimic) is asked to engage in normalized eating, changes in affect are readily apparent. Exaggerated anger regarding "being watched all of the time" (typically referring to observations while eating, or after a meal), unit rules (if the patient is an inpatient), and being "forced" to eat "unreasonable" (i.e., normal) amounts of food is common. Increases in anxiety or depressive symptomatology are also often seen. The patient's behavior and affect when placed on a consistent meal plan of normal food portions can provide an objective index of the severity of the eating disorder. If the person becomes very emotional and/or attempts to avoid eating or to engage in purgative habits, the evaluator should strongly suspect the presence of anorexia or bulimia nervosa.

Based upon the fear-related behavior that is associated with "forbidden" foods, Rosen and Leitenberg (1982) have recommended the use of test meals to assist in the diagnosis of individuals who are anorexic or bulimic. Their procedure is similar to the use of behavioral avoidance tests in assessing individuals with anxiety disorders (e.g., obsessive-compulsive disorders, simple phobias). The following case examples illustrate the use of test meals for assessing two resistant patients.

Case Example. Cindy was a 15-year-old female of normal height, 5 ft. 4 in. tall, and low weight, 103 lbs. During the past six months, she had lost approximately 15 lbs. An initial interview with Cindy found that she had begun to vomit junk foods and vigorously exercise every day about six to eight months prior to referral. Three months later, she began to skip meals and was very reluctant to eat with her family. After her parents confronted her about not eating, she began to eat more. Her mood became negativistic and she continued to exercise daily. Presently, Cindy reported no purgative behavior, no fear of weight gain, and no difficulty or discomfort eating high-caloric foods. Initial testing was suggestive of a minimizing tendency on Cindy's part, but it did not provide conclusive evidence of an eating disorder.

Cindy's mother was asked to keep Cindy home from school so that all eating could be directly observed. Cindy came to the clinic at her normal dinner time and was asked to consume a hamburger, french fries, and milkshake from a local fast food restaurant. She was informed that she would not be allowed to use the rest room unsupervised for two hours after the meal. After 45 minutes Cindy managed to eat 20% of her hamburger, 5% of the french fries, and refused to drink the milkshake. After informing Cindy that she would continue to be supervised during and after meals, she admitted her fear of gaining weight and that she was purging via self-induced vomiting after meals. She was referred for out-patient treatment, which targeted elimination of purging, normalization of eating and weight level, and reduction of fear of weight gain.

Case Example. Sheila was an 18-year-old female who had lost approx-imately 20 lbs. during the past five months. She weighed 116 lbs. and was 5 ft. 7 in. tall when she presented for evaluation. Her parents reported that she had been moping around the house ever since her grandfather died last year, and that her eating had gradually deteriorated since that time. She had been very close to her grandfather. Recently she had begun to skip meals entirely. Interview and testing did not support a diagnosis of eating disorder. However, Sheila was reportedly omitting some high-calorie foods from her diet that she "used to enjoy." Following a normal breakfast and lunch, she was invited to eat a test meal of a hamburger, french fries, and milkshake. She was able to eat 100% of the hamburger and fries, and about 80% of the milkshake. Further monitoring at home supported the conclusion that Sheila was not purging, and was able to consume high-calorie foods without distress. However, she reported symptoms of depression, including sad affect, depressed mood, tearful-ness, irritability, sleep problems, loss of appetite, and anhedonia. Testing results, using the Beck Depression Inventory and MMPI, supported her self-report, with a BDI score of 26 and a t-score of 81 on the D scale of the MMPI. Treatment targeted normalized eating and weight level, relief of depression, and stress management/problem solving skills training.

In both case examples, a behavioral test of eating was used to deter-mine the appropriate diagnosis. In the first case example, the patient's behavior and affective reaction to eating was indicative of an eating dis-order. She ate a minimal portion of the test meal and experienced anxiety after eating. In the second case, however, the patient had no difficulty consuming the test meal, and had no subsequent negative emotional reac-tion. This information facilitated ruling out an eating disorder. Therefore, in cases involving a resistant patient, or when diagnosis is not clear, the utilization of a test meal can often provide invaluable information regard-ing the presence or absence of anorexia or bulimia nervosa.

Alternation of Anorexia and Bulimia Nervosa

It has been our experience that bulimics are usually quite secretive about their purgative behavior. They may, as a result of treatment inter-vention, change their technique of purging. For example, an adolescent who vomits may begin to exercise excessively in her room at night, or begin using laxatives or diuretics. Anorexics are much more blatant in displaying their eating disorder, and often manipulate the family by refusing to eat. In order to appease family members, many bulimics and anorexics "change" from anorexia to bulimia and vice versa. As the presenting eating problem is targeted for change, the patient may adopt a different, but no less dangerous, maladaptive eating style to cope with stress. An anorexic may begin to eat in order to please her parents, therapists, and other significant individuals, but begin to purge in order to rid herself of the food. In a similar fashion, a bulimic may become more restrictive about the amount and types of food she consumes as her purging is gradually limited. Therefore, careful monitoring of the patient by family members at home, or hospital staff while the patient is in the hospital, is necessary to insure that this alternation of anorexia and bulimia nervosa is properly recognized and treated. In the following case, an example of this phenomenon is provided.

Case Example. Gina was a 21-year-old who was referred by her family physician. She lived at home with her parents and attended the local university. Gina weighed 105 lbs. at initial assessment and was 5 ft. 7 in. tall. She had been at her current weight level for six months, after losing approximately 30 lbs. on a liquid diet. She reported that she felt no desire to continue losing weight, but did not want to gain any weight. She reportedly ate three times per day, and denied all symptoms of anorexia during the initial interview, with the exception of amenorrhea. Her testing results were indicative of minimization of problems, with all scores in the normal range. Her MMPI was invalid, suggesting a "fake good" profile. Purging via vomiting, laxatives, diuretics, or excessive exercise was denied. No forbidden foods were reported, although the patient reported that she "did not like" a large number of foods, including red meat, sweets, pizza, fried foods, and butter. Her parents reported that Gina did not eat breakfast, and ate very little at dinner, usually asserting that she had already eaten or was not hungry. She reported to her family that she ate her school lunches. However, she rarely ate lunch at home during the weekends.

Gina was asked to eat a test meal of a hamburger, french fries, and a soft drink (nondiet). She ate 30% of the hamburger, 10% of the french fries, and 25% of the soft drink. Upon questioning, Gina reported that these foods caused stomach problems, and that she could not eat any more. After eating, she appeared agitated, and repeatedly asked to leave the room. Based on the information provided by her parents, her response to the test meal, and her low body weight, the patient was hospitalized for treatment of anorexia nervosa.

After three weeks of inpatient treatment, Gina had gained 8 lbs., and she began to complain of "feeling fat" and discomfort during and after eating. After a meal, the patient was found vomiting in a staff bathroom, and, after confrontation, she reported that she had been purging twice a week for the past two weeks. The patient was placed on more strict staff supervision after meals, and treatment emphasis was placed on modification of body image disturbances and elimination of purging via exposure with response prevention.

Recognition of Family Dysfunction

The family members of an eating disorder patient can often be the source of much information about the patient's behavior at home. However, when working with these families, the clinician should be aware of family problems which are typical in eating disorder populations. Family members of these patients often present a distorted perspective of the patient's behavior. This distortion may occur as a result of the family members' lack of knowledge regarding eating disorders, the family's own atypical eating patterns, or the family's perception of why the patient has his/her eating problems.

During the assessment of an eating disordered patient, the family's level of knowledge about eating disorders should be ascertained. Often, the families are misinformed, or hold certain erroneous beliefs about the patient's reason for restrictive eating, purging or overeating. Common misconceptions are the belief that the patient is willfully trying to disrupt family relations, that the parents were not sufficiently attentive in the past, or that there is something inherently wrong with the patient (e.g., a chronic liar or a troublemaker).

The eating patterns of the family should also be evaluated. There is often a parent or sibling who has chronic weight problems, and, as a result, may be a chronic dieter. Modeling of diet conscious behavior can often be detrimental to the patient's recovery. Also, the family may not have modeled healthy eating habits. For example, many families do not eat at specified times as a family unit, but eat individually while watching television, studying, or driving in the car to work or school. Others may prefer foods high in lipids or cholesterol. The family may be somewhat surprised to learn that this pattern of eating is unhealthy, and must be modified in order to facilitate the patient's own behavior change. Resistance to changing the family's eating style is often seen when this topic is broached in the treatment process.

Summary

Assessment of the resistant patient can be an extremely difficult process, and therefore the clinician assessing this type of patient must be aware of the potential problems which may occur. Minimization of symptomatology during the interview and on questionnaires is very common. Also, these patients often provide explanations for their atypical eating habits which sound quite valid, such as a desire to be "healthy" or stomach problems. Such patients often respond to interview questions and questionnaires with a defensive (or minimization) response style. Therefore, behavioral data from test meals, and information from significant others (e.g., parents, siblings, spouse, friends) must be utilized to establish the presence or absence of clinical problems related to eating. Based on use of a test meal and use of significant others in the assessment process, a more accurate diagnosis and appropriate treatment plan usually can be made.

ASSESSMENT OF INPATIENTS

As noted earlier, many resistant patients cannot be evaluated in an unstructured outpatient setting. Therefore, hospitalization is often required for such cases. This section describes the methods used for evaluating these patients in a hospital environment.

Direct Observation of Eating by Hospital Staff

One of the most important functions of a hospital environment is to allow the treatment staff to observe closely the particular problems associated with eating for each patient. In general, direct observation of eating is a useful method for clarifying diagnosis, correcting poor eating style, ensuring accurate recording of food consumption, and preventing the hiding of food during meals.

In the hospital environment, it is relatively easy to expose patients to meals containing a variety of low- and high-calorie foods and to directly observe eating behavior and emotional reactions to eating. As discussed earlier, this approach is particularly useful for diagnosing patients who have been referred for an eating disorder evaluation, but claim to have no problems with eating. The following case example illustrates how direct observation of eating can be used in an inpatient setting. It should be noted that these observations can usually be conducted in an unobtrusive manner by hospital staff. The unobtrusive nature of these observations provides a more naturalistic evaluation of eating behavior than the test meal procedures described in Chapter 3.

Case Example. Stephanie was a 19-year-old patient who was admitted to the hospital for depression and low body weight. During the previous six months she had lost approximately 20 lbs. Her weight upon admission was 98 lbs. and she was 5 ft. 4 in. tall. She was more than 15% underweight and thus met the weight criterion for anorexia nervosa. She denied any fear of weight gain, however, and claimed that her weight loss was due to depression and lack of appetite. The interview revealed some inconsistencies and psychological tests suggested a response style of minimizing her problems. To assist in her diagnosis and to help her gain weight, she was placed on a 2500 kcal/day meal plan which required the consumption of many high-calorie foods. Unobtrusive observation of her eating showed she avoided eating high-calorie foods even following encouragement from the staff to do so. In addition to avoiding these "forbidden" foods, she was also observed hiding food, using napkins to absorb grease from fried foods, taking very small bites of food, and preparing very large salads. It was suspected that Stephanie was engaging in these behaviors because she believed they would prevent weight gain. She was directly confronted with these suspicions and eventually admitted that she strongly feared weight gain. With further encouragement and support from the staff, Stephanie eventually came to accept a diagnosis of anorexia nervosa and she began to comply with the treatment program. To help her begin eating larger amounts of food, her meal plan was reduced to 1200 kcal/day and gradually increased to 2500 kcal/day over the next 10 days.

Direct observation of eating can also be helpful in determining poor eating habits that may contribute to the maintenance of an eating disorder. For obese patients, there are several eating habits that can seriously interfere with consistent dieting. For example, consistent choice of high-caloric foods can hinder the rate of weight loss. Additionally, a fast rate of eating, limited liquids, and consumption of low-calorie foods at the end of the meal are all factors which contribute to greater caloric consumption for an equivalent degree of fullness. These factors can be directly observed during meals and targeted for change if necessary. For anorexics, eating styles tend to be somewhat reversed to those of obese and binge-eating patients. These patients usually eat very slowly, take very small bites, drink large amounts of fluids, and consume low-calorie foods early in the meal. These behaviors are all designed to avoid forbidden foods and/or lower caloric consumption. During meals, these behaviors can be noted and targeted for change during the course of treatment. The following case examples illustrate the use of behavioral observation procedures with inpatients diagnosed as compulsive overeating and bulimia nervosa.

Case Example. Mike was 34 years old at the time of referral to the inpatient eating disorder program for obesity and compulsive overeating. Initially, he was allowed to choose his meals without following a prescribed meal plan. Direct observation showed that Mike frequently chose foods high in calories for his entree and dessert and rarely selected fruit, salads, or lean meats such as fish, chicken, or poultry. During meals Mike was observed to eat very quickly, to take very large bites, and to wait until after eating to drink his beverage. He reported continued hunger following the meal. Based on this information, Mike was placed on a 1500 kcal/day meal for weight reduction and was given practice and feedback to correct the problems with his eating style. The meal plan required Mike to select a wider variety of foods that were more nutritious yet lower in caloric value. Instructions to modify eating style required Mike to drink a large glass of water approximately 30 minutes before each meal, to put his fork down between bites, to chew his food more slowly, and to eat lower calorie foods at the beginning of each meal. Mike found that he could eat a wider variety of foods while feeling satiated and consuming fewer calories.

Case Example. Becky was 15 years old at the time of referral for bulimia nervosa. She was of normal weight (115 lbs.) for her height (5 ft. 3 in.). She reported the typical binging and purging associated with this disorder. She also claimed to have little voluntary control over vomiting. When she thought about the food in her stomach she could vomit without having to physically induce it (e.g., sticking her finger down her throat or contracting abdominal muscles). It was difficult to establish from self-report which foods were most likely to cause this reaction as she reported that even a glass of water could induce vomiting. Hence, it was decided to allow Becky to select foods on her own accord with the encouragement to select from a wide variety of foods so as to obtain adequate nutrition. Becky was closely monitored during meals for food consumption and associated urges to vomit. She was also prevented from using the bathroom for two hours following meals. Direct observation showed that Becky was able to consume a wide variety of fruits and vegetables, diet soft drinks, and low calorie entrees without experiencing significant discomfort or strong urges to vomit. Average daily caloric consumption was calculated to be approximately 1200 kcals. She reported much greater discomfort after consuming high-calorie desserts, snacks, and entrees such as ice cream, cookies, and red meats. Becky's meal plan was subsequently set at 1200 kcals. Foods that were found to cause discomfort and/or urges to purge were designated to be forbidden foods and were gradually incorporated into her meal plan. This meal plan was systematically increased over the next two weeks until Becky was consuming an average of 1800 kcals and maintaining a normal weight (112–117 lbs.).

Another important aspect of directly observing eating is to ensure that an accurate recording of food consumption is being made. In our program, patients are asked to estimate the percentage eaten of each selected food item. The food item and the percentage eaten are both recorded on an inpatient food monitoring/meal plan record such as the one shown in Figure 6.1.

An eating disorder staff member gives them immediate feedback about the accuracy of their recording and initializes the monitoring form for verification. As can be seen in Figure 6.1, this form is used by the patients to plan their meals ahead of time. The process of planning meals is presented in the following subsection. The "foods selected" column of this form is used to record accurately any deviations in the planned meal. Oddities in eating style such as the use of excessive salad dressing, not eating the skin of fried chicken, and so forth can be noted in the comment section for the dietician to consider when calculating caloric consumption. While obese patients may tend to underestimate the amount they have eaten, anorexic and restrictive bulimics frequently overestimate their food consumption. More extreme problem eating behaviors should be directly confronted by the staff during or following the meal. For example, some patients may ask for larger or smaller than normal servings when going through the serving line, while anorexics may hide food under dishes and/or in their napkins. Thus, close examination of each patient's eating behaviors is required to ensure that food consumption is being accurately recorded.

Quantification of Calories

Alteration of abnormal weight levels and poor dietary habits are usually the initial goals of inpatient treatment and require continued attention throughout treatment. Weight gain is particularly important for anorexia and bulimia nervosa cases which are often characterized by dangerously low weight levels and/or poor physical condition due to recurrent binging and purging. In accomplishing these goals, the assessment and quantification of caloric consumption plays a very important role. However, severe eating disorder patients tend to obsess about even small changes in weight or eating habits. Therefore, care must be taken to obtain information about caloric consumption in such a way as to minimize the obsessiveness in these patients.

In our program, we have found that the use of a dietary exchange system, rather than calories, serves as an adequate method for planning meals and measuring food consumption. The implementation of this system requires patients to attend a separate group that has been designed specifically for the purpose of planning meals and learning about nutrition. An eating disorder therapist and a registered dietician are present to instruct the patients in selecting foods to meet their required exchanges.

Inpatient Meal Plan and Food Monitoring Record

NAME __John B.__
DATE __3-3-89__
DOCTOR __R. Snyder__

Eating Disorder Meal Plan Record

PLANNED MEAL	FOODS SERVED/CHOSEN	AMOUNT EATEN %	CALORIES	COMMENTS	INITIALS OF PERSON RECORDING
Breakfast: Fruit Juice Scrambled Eggs Sausage Bread	Fruit Juice ——— Scrambled Eggs — Bacon ——— Toast ———	100% 100% 80% 100%		Pt. had to switch bacon for sausage	E.R.
Snack:					
Lunch: Trout Hush Puppies Green Beans Milk	Trout ——— Hush Puppies — Green Beans — Milk ———	100% 100% 100% 100%			J.C.
Snack:					
Dinner: Beef Stroganoff w/noodles Green Peas Cabbage Roll	Beef Stroganoff — Green Peas ——— Cabbage ——— Roll ———	100% 75% 100% 60%		Pt. was upset & reported poor appetite	J.C.
Snack:					
			TOTAL =		

DIETICIAN'S COMMENTS: Pt. is eating according to prescribed meal plan

__Janice B. Callaway, RDE__
Signature of dietician computing calories   Date

FIGURE 6.1. Meal plan and food monitoring record for inpatients.

110

These foods are then listed on an eating disorder food consumption/meal plan form such as the one presented in Figure 6.1. The patients refer to this form when selecting foods at mealtime. After meals, the patients are required to record the foods that were actually chosen and the percentages eaten of each. This information is verified by a staff member and later used by the dietician to calculate the number of calories each patient has consumed for the day. Based on the exchange system, caloric consumption can be estimated as follows:

1 starch exchange = 80 kcals
1 meat exchange (1 ounce) = 55 kcals (lean), 75 kcals (medium fat), or 100 kcals (high fat)
1 vegetable exchange = 25 kcals
1 fruit exchange = 60 kcals
1 milk exchange = 90 kcals (skim), 120 kcals (low fat), or 150 kcals (whole)
1 fat exchange = 45 kcals

The advantage of having the patients use exchanges to plan meals, rather than calories, is that the unit of measurement is less specific and, thus, less likely to promote rigid obsessiveness. In addition, the number of required exchanges in each food group can be altered periodically so as to promote flexibility in food selection without sacrificing nutrition or caloric consumption. For example, a prescribed meal plan may require a patient to eat 6 protein exchanges, 7 starch exchanges, 4 fruits, 2 vegetables, 1 milk, and 3 fats. Later in the program this meal plan can be changed to require the consumption of 5 protein exchanges, 6 starches, 3 fruits, 2 vegetables, 2 milks, and 5 fats. Required caloric consumption can be determined in staffings and presented to the patient in the form of exchanges. During meal planning sessions, these exchanges are presented to the patients on a meal planning card such as the one shown in Figure 6.2. This card is completely laminated with specially coated spaces for writing the required number of each exchange in pencil. Thus, required exchanges can be easily altered to promote a change in caloric consumption or to avoid the development of rigidity in the patient.

Another advantage of using an exchange system is that it promotes proper nutrition in addition to adequate caloric consumption. Poor dietary habits are generally a function of irrational fears associated with certain foods and of the numerous sources of misinformation that exist in the popular literature. If these habits are not corrected, changes in some of the more obvious areas of an eating disorder (e.g., frequency of binging and purging, total caloric consumption) may result in a reduction in adequate nutrition (Kirkley, Agras, & Weiss, 1985).

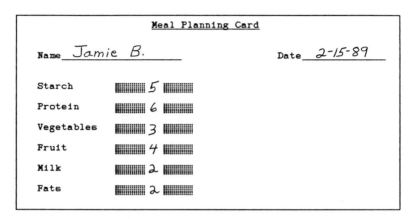

FIGURE 6.2. Example of a meal planning card.

Measurement and Interpretation of Weight Changes

In treating eating disorder patients, one of the first decisions is whether to allow a patient to see his or her weight during treatment. For anorexics and bulimics, it is often very frightening to directly observe increases in weight after they have eaten normal-sized meals and/or forbidden foods. Likewise, it can be demoralizing for an obese patient to follow a strict regimen of eating and exercising and observe only a 1 lb. weight loss at the end of a week. Although these patients may be counseled with regard to appropriate weight levels and rates of weight change, the fine discriminations produced by a scale allow for the development of obsessions about weight gain and compulsive weighing habits. Often, patients report weighing themselves as many as ten times per day before treatment. This type of behavior must not be reinforced by the treatment program, and not allowing direct knowledge of weight level can often modify both the obsessional and behavioral habits.

Generally, anorexics and bulimics exhibit the greatest degree of fear and obsessiveness about weight changes, especially at the beginning of treatment. Our response to this problem is to require these patients to weigh with their back to the scale so that they cannot directly observe their weight level. They are given feedback about their weight, but the feedback is less specific than that provided by a scale calibrated to .25 lbs. For example, a patient may be told where his or her weight is with respect to some previously agreed upon weight range. This feedback gives patients general feedback about weight level without setting the occasion for obsessing about minor weight fluctuations. As treatment progresses and acceptance of more appropriate weight levels improves, patients can be given more specific information about weight changes. Patients who react less emotionally to weight changes are allowed to see their weight while they are being weighed. Consistent weighing under stable conditions (e.g., same time of day, same clothing, and so forth) helps these patients to dispel irrational beliefs and fears about weight change and dietary consumption.

Because weight is such an important concern for eating disorder patients, it is a major focus during treatment planning. In making decisions regarding weight, one must refer to the energy balance model. As noted in Chapter 1, there are 3500 calories in 1 lb. of adipose tissue. Thus, if an individual consumes 3500 calories more than he or she expends (through basal metabolism, exercise, etc.), then that individual will gain 1 lb. of adipose tissue. This model is thoroughly explained to the patients before treatment, and referenced during treatment as their weight changes. In this way, patients can learn that there are long-term patterns of weight change that can be predicted if caloric consumption and physical activity are held constant.

The usual procedure is to estimate (based on factors such as height, weight, sex, age, activity level, etc.) the average daily caloric consumption that would be required to maintain a given individual's weight. A meal plan is then prescribed in order to achieve the desired rate of weight change, whether it be gradual weight loss, weight gain, or weight maintenance. Daily caloric intake and periodic weight changes are charted together and used in making treatment decisions. The form used in charting caloric intake and weight is presented in Figure 6.3.

In Figure 6.3, it can be seen that the patient's weight upon admission was approximately 15 lbs. below an ideal weight for her height. This patient evidenced significant distress at the prospect of weighing more than 120 lbs. Therefore, it was decided to set an initial weight range goal of 115–120 lbs., which resulted in greater cooperation from the patient. By examining the patterns of caloric consumption and weight changes on this form it can be seen that the patient's weight gradually increased as caloric consumption increased. Also, a pattern of restrictive eating became apparent during the first two weekends. Thus, the patient was advised of this restriction and steps were taken to increase compliance with the meal plan. Careful attention to weight changes in the context of the energy balance model can be a useful technique for gauging treatment goals and for detecting patient noncompliance. The following case examples describe how the energy balance model can be used for these purposes.

Case Example. Susan was a 24-year-old obese female receiving inpatient treatment for compulsive overeating and major depression. Her height was 5 ft. 4 in. and her weight upon admission was 198 lbs. The dietician calculated that Susan would require approximately 2200 kcals

<u>**Daily Caloric Intake and Weight**</u>

Name_ Betty F._____   Admission Date_1-22-89

Admission Weight_109 lbs.___   Admission Height_5'5"_

Ideal Body Weight_124 lbs.___   Goal Weight_115-120 lbs._

DATE:	MON	TUES	WEDS	THURS	FRI	SAT	SUN	TOTAL KCALS	AVG KCALS
CALORIES	875	915	1316	1250	1489	1011	1342	8198	1171
WEIGHT	109		108.5		108				

DATE:	MON	TUES	WEDS	THURS	FRI	SAT	SUN	TOTAL KCALS	AVG KCALS
CALORIES	1453	1671	1531	1802	1837	1223	1359	10876	1554
WEIGHT	108.5		108		109				

DATE:	MON	TUES	WEDS	THURS	FRI	SAT	SUN	TOTAL KCALS	AVG KCALS
CALORIES	1882	2026	1983	2334	2181	2468	2201	15075	2153
WEIGHT	109.5		110		111.25				

DATE:	MON	TUES	WEDS	THURS	FRI	SAT	SUN	TOTAL KCALS	AVG KCALS
CALORIES	2352	2675	2409	1915	2314	2475	2500	16640	2377
WEIGHT	112		113.5		113				

DATE:	MON	TUES	WEDS	THURS	FRI	SAT	SUN	TOTAL KCALS	AVG KCALS
CALORIES	2675	2428	2805	2726	2931	2606	2785	18956	2708
WEIGHT	113.5		114		113.75				

FIGURE 6.3. Summary of daily caloric intake and weight changes.

per day to maintain her present weight. Therefore, it was determined that she could lose approximately 2 lbs. per week by consuming 1200 kcals per day. Daily caloric intake and weekly weight changes were recorded and analyzed. By the end of her second week in the program, Susan proudly announced that she had lost 6 lbs. Although the staff were supportive and encouraging of this achievement, they reminded Susan that throughout her treatment she would most likely average about 2 lbs. of weight loss per week and that some of her initial weight loss was probably a result of fluid loss. As predicted, Susan's weight loss over the next two weeks equaled only 2.5 lbs., but during the following week her weight decreased by an additional 1.5 lbs. Over a five-week period Susan consumed a daily average of 1223 kcals and lost 10 lbs. Through this period Susan was able to see that fluctuations in her weight and changes in the rate of weight loss did not effect the long-term trend of weight loss that was predicted by the energy balance model.

Case Example. Cynthia was 21 years old upon admission to the hospital for treatment of bulimia nervosa. Her admission weight was within the normal range for her age and height, but Cynthia made it clear that she did not consider it to be normal. She claimed to feel very overweight and stated that she needed to lose at least 20 lbs. Initially, Cynthia was placed on a low calorie 1200 kcal/day meal plan to give her time to adjust to eating full meals. As expected, her weight decreased a few pounds during the first week and a half and Cynthia was happy with the treatment program. However, Cynthia was then placed on a weight maintenance meal plan of 1800 kcals per day. The following week, her weight loss ceased and she experienced a gain in weight of half a pound. Cynthia was not happy with this occurrence, but she continued to follow her meal plan. Remarkably, her weight began to decrease again despite her apparent consumption of 1800 kcals per day. This unexplained weight loss prompted further assessment of the situation. A random room search was conducted and Cynthia was observed more closely during meals. It was discovered that Cynthia was hiding food during meals. Also, Cynthia's roommate reported that she saw Cynthia exercising in her room late one night. Thus, Cynthia received unit restrictions and close supervision when not in therapy. Eventually, Cynthia was able to become more accepting of her weight and learned that she could maintain her weight while eating a wide variety of foods in healthy quantities.

Another common problem regarding weight change is that of increasing weight in some anorexic patients who have never been overweight. A history of constant thinness suggests that these individuals may have been destined to be somewhat thin even without the influence of anorexic eating habits. Furthermore, there is evidence which suggests that chronic overfeeding can result in elevated metabolic rates and, in turn, slower rates of weight gain for an equivalent number of calories (Apfelbaum, Bostsarron, & Lacatis, 1971; Apfelbaum, 1975; Miller, 1975). We have had patients who were eating over 3000 kcal/day and not gaining weight. It was necessary for these patients to eat between 3500–4000 kcal/day before consistent weight gain could be obtained. In most cases, however, a diet of at least 3000 calories will be required to achieve weight gain in anorexics and low-weight bulimics. Consider the following case example.

Case Example. Amy was an 11-year-old anorexic. She was 4 ft. 10 in. tall and weighed 78 lbs. Although there was evidence of obesity in her immediate family, Amy was always a small child and was never overweight. Refeeding began at 1500 kcals per day and was systematically increased by 300 kcals every two days until Amy was consuming an average of 3000 kcals per day. At this point Amy had gained 5 lbs. However, despite prohibited exercise and complete compliance with the meal plan, Amy's weight ceased to increase during the next three weeks. Thus it was necessary to raise her meal plan further. It was only after Amy was eating 3600 kcals per day that she was able to achieve a consistent weight gain of 1 to 2 lbs. per week.

Changes in a patient's body weight are very important to both the patient and to the treatment staff. Therefore, it is important to be able to account for these changes in a systematic and understandable fashion. For the patient, interpreting weight changes in the context of the energy balance model provides understanding and a sense of control over weight. For the treatment staff, the energy balance model is an essential tool for interpreting weight changes and planning treatment goals.

Detection of Purgative Behavior

The most common forms of purging used by anorexics and bulimics include self-induced vomiting, laxative and diuretic abuse, and excessive exercise. While purging can occur at any time of the day or night, these patients usually attempt to purge shortly after eating to relieve anxiety and to decrease the change of weight gain. Thus, in our program, patients are placed under close observation for two hours following each meal. After two hours, most of the food ingested will have been absorbed by the body and purgative behaviors will have little effect on changes in weight. During this two-hour period, patients are allowed to go to the bathroom only with supervision. Patients are encouraged to use the bathroom prior to mealtime.

Purging may also take the form of excessive exercise. Patients who are prone to excessive exercise will take every opportunity to engage in physical activity. We have had patients wake up at night to exercise in their room, run through the hallways and up and down stairways when unobserved, and run vigorously when allowed to go outside for a walk in the hospital courtyard. Thus, mild, therapeutic exercise (e.g., slow walking) is often allowed, but only with the direct supervision of an eating disorder attendant. In addition, exercise is not allowed within two hours after a meal as this can be experienced by the patient as an anxiety-reducing behavior and can maintain exercise as a purgative habit.

Finally, some patients may buy laxatives and diuretics while on pass and sneak them into the hospital. To discourage this, the patients must be informed that their rooms will be randomly searched for such products. If such items are found, patients may be prohibited from taking a therapeutic pass on the following weekend, they may be given room restriction, or other unit privileges can be revoked. Because it is impossible to account for all of an individual's behavior even in the hospital, it is important for the patient to understand that there will be immediate and meaningful consequences for continued eating disorder behavior.

Summary

Assessment of the resistant eating disorder patient is a difficult process at best. However, the structure of a hospital environment allows for a greater degree of control in the assessment of these patients. The assessment techniques which particularly lend themselves to the hospital environment include: (1) direct observation of eating; (2) precise quantification of caloric consumption; (3) careful measurement and interpretation of weight changes; and (4) detection of purgative behaviors.

Chapter 7
Atypical Eating Disorders and Other Problems of Eating

Very little attention has been given to defining and describing atypical eating disorders. The third edition of the *Diagnostic and Statistical Manual of Mental Disorders* (American Psychiatric Association, 1980) gave little clarification for this class of disorders. The criteria were described as: "a residual category for eating disorders that cannot be adequately classified in any of the previous categories" (p. 73). Thus, researchers and clinicians could diagnose any problem which did not fit the specific criteria for other eating problems as an atypical eating disorder. Additional guidelines have been included in the revised edition (DSM-III-R, APA, 1987) and specific examples were provided. The categories described in the manual include: (1) a person of average weight who does not have binge-eating episodes but frequently engages in self-induced vomiting for fear of gaining weight; (2) all of the features of anorexia nervosa in a female except absence of menses; and (3) all of the features of bulimia nervosa except the frequency of binge-eating episodes. Each of the categories described in the DSM-III-R will be addressed separately under the section labeled "Atypical Eating Disorders." In addition, differential diagnosis of eating disorders from other disorders which involve disturbed eating patterns will be addressed in the section labeled "Eating Problems that Resemble Eating Disorders." This distinction is made to illustrate which types of eating problems should be classified as atypical eating disorders and which types of eating problems should be classified as other psychiatric diagnoses.

ATYPICAL EATING DISORDERS

Bulimia without Binge-Eating Episodes

According to the DSM-II-R (American Psychiatric Association, 1987, p. 68), binge eating must be defined as "rapid consumption of a large amount of food in a discrete period of time." A number of individuals who purge in order to regulate weight have never engaged in binge eating which fits this description. There appears to be a high degree of variability in what each patient considers to be a "binge" or what intake is sufficient to warrant purging. For example, we have seen many "bulimics" who purge via self-induced vomiting after eating any amount of food which they believe will produce weight gain. For example, purging may follow a "binge" involving two Hershey's kisses. However, this same individual may consume a large baked chicken breast, baked potato, and tossed salad and refrain from purging. On the other hand, many "bulimics" feel they must purge if they eat a snack, such as a cookie, as opposed to a meal. Our experience indicates that each patient has developed idiosyncratic rules which determine whether or not the intake is "bad" or "fattening" and should be purged. The current diagnostic criteria prohibit a diagnosis of bulimia nervosa for the patient who is purging but does not binge, defined as consumption of large quantities of food. These cases typically display symptoms of anorexia and bulimia nervosa, but do not meet the DSM-III-R criteria for either disorder. The following case examples illustrate how such cases should be evaluated and conceptualized.

Case Example. Tina was a 17-year-old senior in high school. She was referred for evaluation of her eating behavior by her school guidance counselor. The counselor had recently learned that she was vomiting nearly every day. The counselor had observed Tina's eating behavior at lunch and reported that she had not noticed Tina avoiding high-calorie foods or eating large amounts. She also reported that Tina denied episodes of binge eating but was willing to admit that she vomited to help control her weight.

Tina was evaluated via clinical interview, self-report instruments, behavioral observation, and self-monitoring for her caloric intake. Height and weight measurement indicated that Tina was 5 ft. 7 in. tall and weighed 123 lbs. During the interview Tina admitted to feeling overweight and to vomiting on a daily basis for over six months. She denied episodes of binge eating, stating that she had not eaten over 400 calories per meal (1200 per day) since she started high school. Tina also denied avoidance of any particular foods although she stated that she preferred chicken and fish to red meats. Body image assessment using the BIA indicated body image distortion (T score for CBS = 70) as well as an extreme preference for thinness (T score for IBS = 18). Scores of 102 and 35 on the BULIT and the EAT, respectively, indicated that Tina scored within the clinical range for both bulimic and anorexic symptoms. Observation of Tina's eating showed that she did not eat excessively or avoid all high-calorie foods. In addition, her self-monitoring data was consistent with her self-report of purging after consuming forbidden foods, which in her case included chocolate, fried foods, and red meats.

Although Tina did not meet the diagnostic criteria for bulimia nervosa due to the absence of binge-eating episodes, she clearly had severe body image disturbances, particularly a strong preference for thinness, as well as daily purging via self-induced vomiting. Tina was given a diagnosis of Atypical Eating Disorder and was treated via cognitive-behavioral group treatment for bulimia nervosa, with special emphasis on fear of weight gain, body image disturbances, and reduction of purging.

The DSM-III-R criteria also indicate that an individual must engage in a *minimum* average of two binge-eating episodes per week for at least three months. Again, it is our experience that many "bulimics" restrict their intake until they "lose control" and binge. This may occur only once per month but when it does it involves rapid consumption of large quantities of food. This type of patient is also in need of intensive treatment because the restrictive eating, binging, and purging are behavioral manifestations of fear of weight gain and preoccupation with body size, central features of anorexia and bulimia nervosa. The following case example illustrates this type of patient as well.

Case Example. Barb was a 25-year-old kindergarten teacher. She was born in a large city and had moved to start a teaching job approximately one year prior to presentation. Barb had never been away from home for more than two weeks and she readily admitted to feeling homesick. She began eating sweets on weekend evenings when she was working on lesson plans for her students. She did not experience much guilt about this behavior until approximately four months prior to presentation when she was weighed by her gynecologist. She had gained over 10 pounds in one year, and she was cautioned to "get control over the weight" before she gained too much. Barb stated that she had weighed 122 lbs. for most of her adult life (at 5 ft. 5 in. tall) but had weighed 133 lbs. at the doctor's office. She agreed to watch her snacking and to "get out and exercise a little more." She started by joining the YWCA on her way home and by cooking a nutritious meal for her dinner. However, Barb began "craving" sweets on the weekends. She would go to a nearby market and spend over an hour deciding what to buy. She would typically buy only one candy bar or one bag of chips. However, Barb admitted to "losing control" about once per month at which time she would buy as much food as her pocket money would allow. On these occasions Barb would become very depressed and experience tremendous guilt over her behavior. She became preoccupied with thoughts of food during the day and found it difficult to concentrate on her lesson plans. By the time Barb presented for treatment, she had begun taking laxatives every night to control her weight.

Barb was diagnosed as Atypical Eating Disorder since she did not binge as often as twice per week. She did engage in purgative habits, however, and was preoccupied with body size. She was referred for cognitive-behavioral group therapy with special emphasis on stimulus control procedures as well as cessation of laxative abuse. She was also seen individually for problems related to low self-esteem and depression.

Subclinical Anorexia

We have seen many patients with anorexic symptoms that are less severe than those required for diagnosis of anorexia nervosa. In particular, many young adolescent females have been referred because of extreme dietary practices or desire to lose weight, although they have lost less than 15% body weight or have not ceased menstruating. These individuals are at high risk for developing anorexia and/or bulimia and should be evaluated for treatment even in the absence of the full clinical syndrome. Many of these cases of subclinical anorexia are simply patients who are referred soon after the symptoms of anorexia develop. Our clinical experience suggests that the prognosis for these subclinical anorexics is much better than that of more chronic cases. Therefore, early and intense treatment of these cases may be very important to prevent the more intractable syndrome of anorexia nervosa from fully developing.

A note of caution should be made at this point as the potential for "creating" an anorexic or bulimic exists when the subclinical patient is treated in a group format with more "seasoned" eating disorder patients. The content of group therapy discussions as well as informal communication among the patients may provide "new ideas" for weight control for the younger, more naive patient. A case example is provided to illustrate this point.

Case Example. Mary was a 12-year-old girl who had just completed the seventh grade. She had lost 7 pounds in a two-month period and her mother was concerned about her restricted eating. Mary denied binge eating or any attempts to control her weight by vomiting, laxatives, diuretics, or excessive exercise. In fact, she appeared surprised when asked about laxatives as a means of weight control. She denied wanting to lose weight but refused to consider gaining "even 1 pound." Mary's responses to the body image assessment did not indicate that she viewed herself as being overweight, nor did she desire to be very thin. However, an interview with Mary's parents indicated that she weighed herself several times per day and that she became very upset if her friends weighed less than she did.

Observation of Mary's eating behavior found that she ate very small portions and restricted her food choices to lean meats and vegetables. When given a test meal, Mary refused to eat the high-calorie foods presented.

An overall analysis of Mary's assessment data indicated that she was overly concerned with weight and refused to maintain a normal weight for her age and height. Although she did not admit to a strong preference for thinness, her eating behavior and her behavior in the home indicated a definite body image disturbance. Mary was diagnosed with subclinical anorexia as she had not lost sufficient weight at the time of assessment to warrant a diagnosis of anorexia nervosa. Also, she had not ceased menstruation.

Mary was referred to group therapy for her eating problems. This group included other anorexics and bulimics. After one treatment meeting, however, it was the recommendation of the group therapist that Mary receive individual rather than group treatment. This decision was made when Mary began asking another patient for "tips" on laxative abuse. She was overheard asking which types were most effective, how many to take, and when to take them for the most convenience. It was feared that Mary might become more sophisticated at maladaptive means of weight control (e.g., laxatives) as a result of being treated with a group of bulimia and anorexia nervosa patients who had long histories of food refusal, purging via self-induced vomiting and laxatives, and compulsive exercise. Although most individuals are aware of the many maladaptive means of weight control, the younger, subclinical patient may learn more maladaptive behaviors as a function of being treated in a group format. For these reasons, she was removed from the group and treated individually.

Atypical eating disorders may be as pathological as bulimia nervosa or anorexia nervosa. Individuals with idiosyncratic dietary rules or maladaptive means of weight control in the absence of binge eating may be atypical or they may be in the early stages of developing an eating disorder. In the case of the latter, it is very important to identify the problem early so that treatment may be initiated as quickly as possible. An extensive assessment battery, including test meals, self-monitoring, psychological test data, body image assessment, and interviews with significant others, is often necessary to determine the degree to which the individual is cooperating and giving an accurate self-report. It is important to remember that individuals with recent onset of the disorder may not have sufficient insight and may be unaware of their problems to a certain degree. Others may fear negative evaluation from the interviewer or family/friends if they acknowledge their problems. Proper diagnosis and conceptualization is very important for individual treatment planning as each patient may require different elements of the treatment package for successful treatment. This issue is particularly important with atypical eating disorder patients as their behaviors may be very idiosyncratic and require novel or creative treatment approaches.

EATING PROBLEMS THAT RESEMBLE EATING DISORDERS

Differential diagnosis of eating disorders from other disorders that involve disturbances in eating patterns or weight level can be very difficult at times. Cases which involve vomiting or food refusal in the absence of body image disturbance can be particularly difficult to diagnose. A large number of alternative diagnoses must be considered and tested systematically to rule out medical and psychiatric disorders. Denial of body image disturbance must also be considered as many patients are unwilling to admit to self-perpetuation of the eating problem. A case example is provided to exemplify differential diagnosis of potential disorders or problems that may mimic an eating disorder such as bulimia nervosa.

Case Example. Tanya was a 21-year-old female who presented to the Eating Disorders Clinic with chief complaints of nausea, vomiting, and feelings of extreme bloatedness. She had undergone a series of medical evaluations which failed to identify a medical basis for the nausea or vomiting. Tanya denied that the vomiting was "self-induced"; rather she stated that she often "vomited automatically" after eating. When asked if only certain foods caused her to get sick, she replied that eating too much or eating foods such as sweets or dairy products have often caused her to feel sick or vomit.

Tanya weighed 115 lbs. and was 5 ft. 6 in. tall. When asked if she had ever attempted to lose weight by vomiting she stated "no, I don't want to gain weight but I don't really need to lose either." Tanya reported that her highest weight level was 125 lbs. in her senior year of high school. She was now at her lowest weight, 114 lbs. She denied ever feeling more than mildly dissatisfied with her figure or her weight.

Further questioning showed that Tanya had also experienced episodes of muscle weakness and fatigue, as well as joint pain and tingling sensations in her extremities. Dizziness and chest pain were described on days when vomiting occurred. Tanya noted that she had fainted on two occasions when she stood up after vomiting. Menstrual irregularities were described with complaints of both absence of menstrual flow and extremely heavy flow. Tanya described a fair amount of pain associated with heavy periods. Alcohol and drug abuse were denied although Tanya did admit to "sipping a little whiskey" on occasion. She also described taking a number of over-the-counter medications such as Tylenol and other pain relievers. Social history indicated a mild level of anxiety with members of the opposite sex and little desire to engage in physical contact of a sexual nature.

Tanya's clinical presentation was somewhat atypical of bulimia nervosa in that she denied a desire to manage her weight through vomiting as well as a desire to lose weight. However, initial interviews are often insufficient to completely assess the individual's body image disturbance as the patient may have little insight or be unwilling to discuss her fears related to weight. Careful examination of Tanya's symptom presentation suggested the possibility of a somatization disorder. Tanya described four gastrointestinal symptoms, one pain-related symptom, three cardiopulmonary symptoms, two conversion or pseudoneurologic symptoms, two sex-related symptoms, and three symptoms related to the reproductive system. It is interesting to note, however, that each of the symptoms described were common to bulimia nervosa. Suspecting somatization disorder, we requested Tanya' medical records. They showed that she had been to the community free clinic on twelve occasions in the three months prior to presentation and had expressed a number of additional symptoms, such as headaches and blurred vision. This combination of symptoms satisfied the DSM-III-R criteria for somatization disorder. In addition, the records showed that she was well-known by community physicians as a result of numerous unsuccessful attempts to secure pain medication. Thus, it seemed likely that Tanya presented to the Eating Disorders Clinic in an attempt to secure medication for her physical symptoms. She was confronted with this formulation and angrily withdrew from the evaluation. A cursory examination of her presenting problem may have led to an incorrect diagnosis of bulimia nervosa and inappropriate treatment.

Affective Disorders

Anorexia and bulimia nervosa patients often present with complaints of depressed mood as well as neurovegetative symptoms such as appetite/sleep disturbance, weight loss, decreased interest in sex, and amenorrhea. Differential diagnosis is typically based on the presence or absence of a body image distortion, preference for thinness, and/or fear of weight gain. Carlson and Cantwell (1980) found that although anorexic adolescents described dysphoric mood, low self-esteem, hopelessness, and suicidal ideation, their global ratings of depression were significantly less than those of adolescents with primary affective disorder. The differential diagnosis becomes more difficult when an anorexic patient presents with dysphoric mood, loss of interest, and an appetite disturbance with subsequent weight loss. With this type of patient the presence of a body image disturbance and fear of weight gain may be the critical factor in differential diagnosis.

We typically administer a Beck Depression Inventory (BDI) and a Center for Epidemiological Studies Depression Inventory (CES-D) to every individual upon presentation. In addition, the structured interview for secondary psychopathology (see Chapter 5) is administered. Although the incidence of affective disorders is high in bulimia nervosa and anorexia nervosa patients, it is important to identify a primary diagnosis of depression prior to treatment planning. The experienced clinician will remember, however, that cognitive disturbances and low self-esteem may be the result of starvation in the anorexic and a diagnosis should be delayed until the patient has been fed, if possible. We have found that test meals (Rosen et al., 1985) can often provide valuable information regarding fear of weight gain, which aids in the differential diagnosis of depression and anorexia nervosa. A case example is provided to illustrate this assessment strategy.

Case Example. Julie was 23 years old, an English major at a local university. She was very interested in the arts and spent a great deal of her spare time learning ballet. Her family was quite wealthy and, thus, she enjoyed the finer things in life since early childhood. Julie described herself as "happy and content" until approximately three months prior to presentation for assessment of anorexia nervosa. She had sprained her ankle at a football game and had been unable to practice ballet for over two months. She began to lose interest in her school work, her appetite was poor, and few activities were enjoyable. Although Julie had been slightly underweight most of her life, she began losing weight fairly quickly. She presented at a weight level approximately 15% below a normal weight for her height. Julie described her mood as irritable and she admitted to feeling confused and unable to concentrate. She denied actively attempting to diet as well as any maladapative means of weight control. Instead, she reported, "I just don't care about eating anymore, or anything for that matter."

A comprehensive evaluation was undertaken to make a differential diagnosis between major depression and anorexia nervosa. Julie's score on the BDI (32) indicated significant depressive symptomology. Her scores on the eating disorder related questionnaires were far below the cutoffs for bulimia (BULIT = 64) or anorexia nervosa (EAT = 20). Body image assessment indicated that Julie viewed herself as thin (T = 42) and preferred to be slightly underweight (T = 43). In addition, no evidence of body size dissatisfaction was noted. A test meal helped to make the differential diagnosis. Julie was asked to consume a meal consisting of beef, cooked vegetables, tossed salad with dressing, french fries, and two small buttered rolls. An eating disorder patient would be expected to avoid eating large amounts of the high-calorie foods. Julie, in contrast, ate only the buttered rolls and french fries, foods which are not suggestive of a strong fear of weight gain. In addition, she rated her anxiety as low both before and after eating. She also noted that she was not hungry and that the foods had little "taste."

Julie was given a provisional diagnosis of major depression and returned to her previous weight level while receiving treatment for depression, including antidepressant medication and cognitive-behavior therapy. Depressive symptoms were monitored continuously and disturbances in appetite abated as depression improved.

The critical factors in differential diagnosis of eating disorders and affective disorders are related to body image disturbances as well as avoidance of "forbidden" foods. A structured test meal has proved to be a viable assessment strategy to test for the presence of these characteristics. The test meal requries that the patient eat a variety of foods, which typically reveals a significant fear of weight gain. On the other hand, a depressed patient with a poor appetite is less likely to differentially avoid high-calorie foods or show extreme anxiety when presented with high-calorie foods.

Schizophrenia or Psychosis

Earlier conceptualizations of anorexia nervosa considered it to be a variant of schizophrenia because the symptoms of bizarre eating patterns and refusal to eat had the appearance of psychotic behavior. However, the reasons why a schizophrenic refuses to eat are substantially different from those of the anorexic. The schizophrenic or psychotic individual typically refuses to eat due to delusional ideas about the food itself or what the food will do to his or her body. For instance, the paranoid schizophrenic may fear that the food has been poisoned or the food will spoil in his stomach. Although body image distortion in the eating disorder patient may reach delusional proportions and resemble psychotic perceptions, the fundamental cognitive disturbances of schizophrenia are not typically found in anorexia or bulimia nervosa. The incidence of an additional diagnosis of schizophrenia in anorexia nervosa patients has been reported to be between 1% and 7% (Dally, 1969; Farquharson & Hyland, 1966; Hsu, Crisp, & Harding, 1979; Hsu, Meltzer, & Crisp, 1981; Theander, 1970).

Differential diagnosis of schizophrenia from bulimia or anorexia nervosa is based primarily on the presence or absence of bizarre delusions. Although an eating disorder patient may give elaborate and somewhat fantastic reasons for avoiding certain foods, she is usually able to identify her fear of weight gain as the basis for the unusual belief. A schizophrenic, on the other hand, is clearly convinced of the reality of the delusion. In addition, schizophrenics will typically report auditory or visual hallucinations as well as thought disturbances. The beliefs of the eating disorder patient are strictly related to eating and fear of weight gain. A case example is provided to illustrate a differential diagnosis between the two disorders.

Case Example. Debbie was a 23-year-old homemaker. She dropped out of school in her senior year to marry her boyfriend after she had become pregnant. They had been married for six years and had two daughters, ages 6 and 3. Debbie had never worked outside of the home and had very little contact with anyone but her husband and children. She presented for treatment of anorexia nervosa at her husband's insistence after she had lost approximately 20 lbs. in the past three months.

Debbie denied any desire to lose weight and that her husband found her to be "too skinny," but was aware of the "thinness" fad. She refused to even try the foods offered in a test meal and her self-monitoring indicated that she consumed only liquids (i.e., soft drinks and juice). Debbie's husband was largely responsible for the accuracy of the self-monitoring as the patient repeatedly "forgot" to complete the self-monitoring task. He agreed that Debbie had eaten little else but liquids over the past few weeks. He described Debbie as "sort of paranoid" about what she ate and he stated that he had heard the same thing about anorexics. He was unable to relate a history of concern about caloric intake or weight; he stated instead that eating had always been one of the few fun things that he and his wife had shared.

Further assessment found that Debbie did not exhibit any signs of body image concerns or fear of weight gain. No evidence of purging via self-induced vomiting, laxatives, diuretics, or compulsive exercise was found. Debbie's fears appeared to be strictly related to eating solid foods. She was somewhat difficult to interview because her answers to questions were often tangential. When questioned about her avoidance of only solid foods, Debbie became very defensive. After pressing her, she stated that God had told her that solid foods were made up of "small little atoms full of radiation" and because of this belief she drank only liquids. She had not told her husband about the message from God as she felt he would not believe her. As the interview progressed, it became clear that Debbie was experiencing a host of delusional ideas as well as auditory hallucinations. She was a classic case of paranoid schizophrenia who had not decompensated to a low level of functioning.

Differential diagnosis of schizophrenia and anorexia nervosa may require interviewing family members or friends. Careful monitoring of the patient's behavior may help to identify the factors maintaining the behavior and help to rule out the presence of an eating disorder. Self-monitoring may be particularly difficult for the schizophrenic, but asking family members to observe and document eating habits can often circumvent this problem.

Obsessive-Compulsive Disorder

The obsessional quality of eating disorder patients has led some researchers to consider anorexia or bulimia nervosa as being similar to obsessive-compulsive disorder (OCD). The basis of both disorders involves the presence of persistent ideas, thoughts, images, or fears of some unrealistic event. In the OCD patient, the fear may be related to germs or a fear of disease while the anorexic and bulimic patient typically fears weight gain. In addition, there is typically some behavioral habit which is used to reduce the anxiety created by the fears in both disorders. In the OCD patient, the response is some type of compulsive ritual, such as cleaning or checking, while in the bulimic or anorexic, "undoing" is typically in the form of purgative habits.

Differential diagnosis of an obsessive-compulsive disorder and an eating disorder is made on the basis of the content of the obsessive thoughts and the nature of the compulsive behavior. According to the DSM-III-R, the diagnosis of OCD cannot be made if the content of the obsession is solely related to food or eating. A case example of a patient seen in our clinic for differential diagnosis of bulimia nervosa and obsessive-compulsive disorder will be provided to illustrate differences between the two disorders.

Case Example. Noreen was a 19-year-old college student. She was referred for treatment of anorexia nervosa because she had slowly lost weight over the past year. She weighed 102 lbs. at 5 ft. 3 in., when she presented for evaluation. Noreen denied actively trying to lose weight and, in fact, stated that she wished she could regain some weight. Body image assessment results were consistent with Noreen's self-report. She chose a current body size which was identical to that chosen by others for her height and weight and an ideal figure slightly larger than her current body image, indicating an absence of body image distortion and preference for thinness. Body size dissatisfaction was evident as Noreen preferred to be slightly larger than she was at the time of presentation.

Noreen was given a test meal to determine the degree to which she would avoid high-calorie foods. She refused to eat even one bite. It was not until after the test meal was completed that Noreen mentioned that she could not eat the foods of the test meal because she had not been able to wash the containers. She explained that she had once noticed a layer of dust on a soup can and that an hour after eating the soup she had become ill. She started thinking about the dust on the can and realized that the can could have been "contaminated." She began thinking of little else and was able to bring food into the house only if she could immediately wash the container in hot water. She was diagnosed as obsessive-compulsive disorder and was treated using exposure with response prevention.

Conversion Disorder or Hysteria

The current DSM-III-R definition of conversion disorder is "a loss of, or alteration in, physical functioning suggesting a physical disorder" (p. 259). In addition, psychological factors are thought to be etiologically related to the symptom and the person must not be conscious of intentionally producing the symptom.

Clinical reports of patients with both anorexia nervosa and hysteria date back to the last century (La Tourette, 1895). Although dual diagnosis of conversion disorder and an eating disorder is relatively uncommon, it is common for an hysterical patient to complain of physical problems related to the gastrointestinal system. Loss of appetite, weight loss, nausea, vomiting, and diarrhea are all common physiological symptoms which are highly affected by psychological conflict or stress.

In the eating disorder patient, the physical symptoms are usually self-induced, such as self-induced diarrhea via laxative abuse. In addition, the anorexic or bulimic typically reports a preference for thinness or a fear of weight gain. In the hysteric, on the other hand, vomiting and weight loss often occur because of the symbolic meaning that food or eating has assumed (Bruch, 1973) or as a result of a traumatic event. In these cases, typical symptoms of eating disorder patients (e.g., body image disturbance) are usually absent. A case example is provided to illustrate this point.

Case Example. Rachel was a 33-year-old single female who was employed as an office clerk. She was referred to the eating disorders unit because she was unable to swallow solids or liquids and was losing weight. The patient lived at home with her parents and had never been married. She described an "unwritten rule" that no one moved out of the house until they were married. The patient had one brother who moved out of the family home when he began college. He was married and living with his wife at the time of Rachel's hospitalization.

Rachel identified the onset of her problems as two years prior when she was feeling stressed on her job due to "sexual harassment." She began having difficulty swallowing and subsequently ate fewer and fewer foods. She had lost approximately 25 lbs. prior to hospitalization and had quit her job due to an increase in fears related to eating.

Rachel underwent a complete medical evaluation but no physical basis could be identified for the problems related to swallowing. A thorough assessment of the patient's history indicated that the fear of choking and/or swallowing dated back to when Rachel was approximately 9 years of age. She developed severe allergies and had required medical attention several times per week. She recalled spending much time with her parents when the other children were out playing. The relationship with her father was described as "unusually close." Although Rachel denied any sexual or physical abuse, observation of interactions with her father during unit visitation prompted the staff to evaluate the situation further. He insisted that she sit on his lap and he continuously stroked her back in an attempt to comfort her. In addition, monitoring of Rachel's food intake indicated a decrease in amount consumed each day she received a visit from her family.

Rachel was interviewed to construct a hierarchy of fears and she quickly identified a fear of "someone forcing something into her mouth" and "not being able to breathe" as her greatest fears. Subsequent sessions with the patient led to an admission of forced oral sex by her father when she was a child. She recalled being left alone for several days after her allergy shots as she was not well enough to eat supper with the family. Further sessions with Rachel found that throughout the years she had many gastrointestinal complaints and avoided intimacy with men due to these physical symptoms. The onset of sexual harassment at work was too stressful for Rachel to deal with assertively and may have been directly related to the onset of problems with swallowing. Although Rachel denied intentionally producing the symptoms, she expressed relief when apprised of her case formulation. Rachel continued to be re-fed while undergoing intensive psychotherapy.

The above case history should illustrate the need for a detailed and comprehensive assessment. It is clear that the patient was unable to cope with the sexual abuse and achieved "primary gain" by keeping the internal conflict out of awareness. The use of desensitization procedures or flooding may have intensified the problem as the fears were based on a realistic stressor.

Garfinkel, Kaplan, Garner, and Darby (1983) described 20 conversion disorder patients who presented with vomiting and or weight loss, but lacked the core features of anorexia or bulimia nervosa. A comparison with 20 anorexia nervosa patients showed that the conversion disorder group had significantly lower scores on the EAT and showed less involvement with dieting on the Restraint Scale. Although the two groups did not differ with regard to weight history, the anorexic group weighed more on presentation than the conversion group. The results of their retrospective analysis showed that patients with conversion disorder had less dissatisfaction with their body parts and their bodies overall, and that they underestimated their body size while anorexics tended to overestimate. With regard to psychological variables, Garfinkel et al. (1983) found that the conversion group had a stronger sense of self-control, less obsessive-compulsive behavior, and more consistent social relationships than the anorexic group. These results should be kept in mind when differential diagnosis of conversion disorder and an eating disorder is required. Body image assessment and questionnaires designed to assess eating disorder pathology (e.g., EAT) are particularly useful in this endeavor. We have seen a number of cases in which specific events in the patient's history appeared to be directly linked to a disturbance of eating. It is often difficult for the patient to identify an event which precipitated the problem or to discuss a traumatic event in the initial evaluation. Therefore, unusual test results and the absence of body image disturbance should alert the clinician to the possibility of a conversion disorder when a person presents with vomiting, problems swallowing, and/or significant weight loss.

Summary

Assessment of eating problems that do not meet the DSM-III-R criteria for bulimia nervosa or anorexia nervosa can be a difficult task. In some cases, the symptoms are indicative of an eating disorder but lack certain symptoms which are considered necessary for diagnosis. In other cases, the symptoms are all present but the level of severity is not sufficient for diagnosis. In both cases, a diagnosis of atypical eating disorder (or eating disorder not otherwise specified) is warranted. In other cases, however, problems related to eating and weight loss are indicative of other psychiatric diagnoses such as affective, anxiety, or conversion disorders.

Very little empirical work has been done in the area of diagnosing atypical eating disorders. Norvell and Cooley (1986) reported on two atypical eating disorder cases which lacked sufficient symptoms for diagnosis of anorexia or bulimia nervosa and concluded that an atypical eating disorder diagnosis was more appropriate than a diagnosis of conversion disorder. Mitchell, Pyle, Hatsukami, and Eckert (1986) reported on 25 cases of atypical eating disorder patients and concluded these cases fell within the general characteristics of anorexia and bulimia nervosa.

There are a number of characteristic behaviors which are critical for diagnosis of anorexia nervosa or bulimia nervosa. In the former, the individual must have experienced sufficient weight loss and refuse to maintain a body weight normal for her height and age. In addition, a body image disturbance must be present and menses absent for at least three months. In the latter, episodes of binge eating must be present and occur frequently. In addition, the individual must engage in some type of purgative behavior, feel a lack of control over eating behavior during binges, and have a persistent overconcern with body shape and weight. Thus, the presence of extreme weight loss, binge eating, and/or purging are necessary for a diagnosis of an eating disorder.

Diagnosis of other problems that involve eating or weight loss may be more difficult. The clinician's assessment of body image disturbance (i.e., body size distortion, preference for thinness, body size dissatisfaction) and fear of weight gain are critical in these cases. Body image concerns and behavioral avoidance of high caloric foods may be the most critical elements of differential diagnosis since these behaviors are much more difficult to disguise than responses to questions during interview or on self-report inventories. We have found that differential diagnosis of these disorders is best conducted by a professional who is familiar with both eating disorders and other medical or psychiatric disorders.

Chapter 8
Treatment Planning and Evaluation

The axiom that psychiatric diagnosis cannot be undertaken for its own sake is certainly applicable for eating disorders. Psychological assessment of eating disorders must relate in some meaningful way to treatment. Thus, this chapter is devoted to relating the previously described assessment procedures to treatment planning, and to the evaluation of treatment. In Table 8.1 the assessment procedures that are recommended as a basic protocol for eating disorders are summarized. Typical problem areas found in eating disorder patients are listed, along with the recommended assessment procedure.

The assessment process should take the clinician about three one- to two-hour sessions. In the third session, there should be enough time to discuss the results of the assessment with the patient, and the recommended treatment plan. In the first session, the patient is administered the structured interview for diagnosis of eating disorders and the Brief Interview of Secondary Psychopathology (BISP). Because the measurement of body image concerns with the BIA is brief, it is recommended that this instrument be administered at each assessment session. Also, height and weight measurement should be taken at all assessment sessions. We recommend that body image assessment be taken before height and weight measurement, because body image can be influenced by weight measurement. After the first session the clinician should have gathered general information regarding the client's eating disorder, and any other significant problems that may be occurring.

If there is time, it is best to administer the BDI, BULIT, EQ-R, and EAT in the first session. Most patients complete these measures in less than 45 minutes. It is best that these measures be interpreted before the next assessment session, as these results may guide subsequent inquiry by the clinician.

Table 8.1. Summary of Suggested Assessment Tools

General Problem Area	Specific Problem	Measure
Eating Disorders	Eating behaviors and cognitions about eating	Structured interview BULIT EQ-R EAT Self-monitoring
	Weight status	Height Weight
	Body image	BIA
Secondary Psychopathology	General screening	BISP
	Depression	BDI
	Anxiety and obsessive-compulsive	STAI MOCI
	Family problems	FES
	Interpersonal sensitivity	FNE
	Personality problems	
		MMPI

In the second session, secondary psychopathology should be assessed. We recommend administering the MOCI, STAI, FES, FNE, and MMPI. The third assessment session should be devoted to reviewing assessment data, case formulation, and discussion of treatment options.

Self-monitoring data is essential to the assessment protocol. We find that two weeks of self-monitoring generally provides a representative sample of the person's eating habits. Thus, the patient should begin self-monitoring immediately after the first session. In the second session, it is wise to begin the session with a review of the client's self-monitoring. In the third session these data can be used to document specific problems of eating and to provide a behavioral analysis of binging, purging, and restrictive eating. Assessment with some patients may take considerably longer, depending on the nature of the problem and time constraints for both clinician and patient.

The following sections describe how assessment results can be used for treatment planning and evaluation. Each of the eating disorders will be discussed, and case examples are presented to illustrate the process of treatment planning and outcome evaluation.

OBESITY AND COMPULSIVE OVEREATING

Much of treatment planning for obese patients will depend on whether there are other psychological or medical problems associated with the eating disorder. If an obese patient with significant secondary psychopathology is treated with a straightforward weight control program, it is likely that treatment will be unsuccessful. Many times weight loss programs have not been successful because of other psychological problems that were not addressed. Thus, it is important to thoroughly assess secondary psychopathology in addition to an individual's eating problems.

The clinician should also evaluate the severity of binge eating when assessing obese patients. Further, the amount of weight that a patient needs to lose is important to consider. If a patient has a significant amount of weight to lose, this may be an immediate health threat that demands immediate intervention. If, on the other hand, a patient is relatively close to goal weight at assessment, this weight may be lost more slowly and treatment planning may need to attend to more weight maintenance issues. The weight history of obese individuals should also be carefully investigated by the assessor. The determination of how a patient has gained weight and how weight is maintained will also have direct treatment implications. It may be that a patient did not gain her weight by ingesting a large amount of calories, but rather her activity has slowly decreased with time. Thus, treatment for this type of case should be more directed at increasing activity level rather than lowering caloric intake.

Case Example. June was single and had recently graduated from law school. She had gained 50 lbs. while at law school, and wished to pursue a weight loss program. Interview data indicated that her eating had become very erratic during law school. Because of spending extensive time in class and with studies, June did not have a regular meal schedule. She often ate while studying, and often ate "on the run." June reported that during this time at law school she rarely sat down to eat a meal. In addition, although June used to ride her bike regularly, during law school she rarely took time to ride her bike except occasionally between semesters. Reportedly, she had not been overweight before this time and had never been on a diet, thus excess weight was reportedly gained while attending law school. It was evident that her weight gain could be attributed primarily to decreased activity rather than increased caloric intake.

The assessment results summarized in Table 8.2 suggested that June had few clinical problems other than obesity. There were no clinical elevations on the MMPI, the BDI score was quite low, and the BISP indicated no significant problems with depression or anxiety. Relatively low scores on the EQ-R and the BULIT suggested that she did not have typical symptoms of bulimia nervosa or compulsive overeating. Because of the absence of secondary psychopathology, she was referred to a standard behavior modification program for treatment of obesity. We recommended this program focus on Energy Balance Training (EBT), a regular meal schedule, increased activities, and stimulus control, as suggested by the treatment plan in Table 8.3. Energy balance training (Johnson & Stalonas,

Table 8.2. Assessment Results

Name: _June S._____ Client #: _B3487_

Eating Disorder Measures: Height: _5'3"_ Weight: _197_ BMI: _36_

EQ-R: _23_ BULIT: _53_ EAT: _15_

BIA: Current: _8 t = N/A_ Ideal: _4 t = N/A_ Difference t-score = _N/A_

Self-monitoring:

Amount Eaten	#	Hunger		Mood		At Home While Eating (%)	Alone While Eating (%)
		Prior	After	Prior	After		
Undereat	6	4	4	3	3	79	100
Normal	9	3	2	2	2	85	75
Slight Overeat	23	4	2	3	3	95	90
Moderate Overeat	8	5	2	3	4	60	60
Binge	0						
Purge	0						

cal/day = 1840   eats/day = 3.29   exercise/day = .14

Secondary Psychopathology:

MMPI Code: _Scale 4 = 62, scale 0 = 63_

Interview Results: Anxiety _3_ Depression _5_

Comments: _no evidence found of mood or anxiety disorders_

BDI: _5_

FNE: _15_

MOCI: Total = _4_ Checking = _1_ Washing = _0_ Slowness = _1_ Doubting = _2_

FES: (t-scores) Cohesion _63_ Expressiveness _42_ Conflict _51_

Independence _49_ Achievement Org. _59_ Intellectual-Cultural Org. _62_

Active _47_ Moral-Religious _50_ Organization _49_ Control _58_

1981) refers to a program which trains the patient in the energy balance model, and also includes stimulus control, meal planning, modification of eating behavior, aerobic exercises, and nutritional training. Also, this approach discourages strict dieting regimes. Regular meal schedules, stimulus control, and increased exercise were particularly appropriate treatment goals for this patient. Primary outcome measures for this patient included the self-monitoring of exercise, amount eaten, and weight loss as measured in pounds and by the Body Mass Index (BMI).

Case Example. Lanny was 28 years old and was working full time at a fast food restaurant. He reported that he had always been somewhat overweight but had gained 70 lbs. in the year prior to treatment. Thus,

Table 8.3. Eating Disorder Treatment Plan

Name: _June S._____ Age: _28_ Sex: _F_

Marital Status: _S._ Occupational Status: _FT, Lawyer_____

A. Problem List: 1. _Obesity_____

2. _Erratic eating_____

B. DSM-III-R Diagnosis:

Axis 1: 316.00, Psychological factors affecting physical cond.

Axis 2: None   Axis 3: Obesity

C. Treatment Plan:

1. Eating Disorder Therapy: _Energy Balance Training,_____
   Regular meal schedule, increase of activities, stimulus_____
   control._____

2. Nutrition Therapy: _Daily Cal.:1200_____

3. Other Problems: _None_____

this patient's weight problem was fairly severe at the time of assessment. A clinical interview found that both Lanny's parents were obese. About one year prior to evaluation Lanny had been promoted to assistant manager of the restaurant at which he was employed. One of the responsibilities of the assistant manager was to close the restaurant at night after all the other employees had left. At the close of each evening, food that had not been served was either thrown away, or the night employees made sure "the food did not go to waste." On almost every evening that he worked, Lanny reported that he ate some food with the other employees, and ate more after they had left for the evening. Thus, Lanny binged most evenings and had done so almost every day for the past year. He reported that he felt "bad about himself" after binging in the restaurant, but that as soon as the last employee left for the evening, he felt compelled to eat. Lanny described his feelings before binging as "uncomfortable." He said that "the pizza was calling him," and that the more he tried to "think himself out of binging" the greater his urges to binge grew. Lanny said that he thought that he binged more at night when he was feeling down. If something was bothering him, or if something upsetting had happened at work, then he was even more likely to binge when others left. Lanny noted that most of his friends were at work, and that when everybody left at night he frequently felt "empty and alone."

Lanny's history suggested that food was very important to him. At home, Lanny reported that food was often used as a reinforcer, or as a way of comforting him. If Lanny was feeling down, his father would often take him to the local ice cream parlor. Lanny noted that he treasured these times, because his father did not spend much time with him doing other activities. He recalled that he was not very popular in grade school. He was always one of the heaviest students in class, which brought positive and negative attention from his peers. In elementary school he and his peers would engage in eating contests—who could eat the fastest and who could eat the most food. This was a contest that Lanny usually won, according to his recollection, and was one of the few activities which consistently produced positive attention from his peers. However, in junior high school, other children began to make fun of his weight and his eating behavior. Thus, Lanny tried to eat little, if anything, for lunch at school. But he recalled that frequently his hunger would "overcome" him, and he would binge on candy in private.

One of the main reasons that Lanny had presented for treatment was that he was quite interested in female companionship. He felt that most women would not go out with him because of his weight. He had never dated much in the past, and exhibited significant apprehension about asking women out for dates.

Lanny's assessment results are summarized in Table 8.4. It was clear that he had other psychological concerns that might negatively interact with treatment for obesity. Lanny's scores on the EQ-R and the BULIT suggested that he had significant problems with compulsive overeating. That the BULIT score was greater than 102 and the EQ-R total score was greater than 40, corroborated a diagnosis of compulsive overeating. Self-monitoring data provided further information concerning the determinants of binge eating. These data showed a relationship between Lanny's mood and his binging behavior, that is, negative affect consistently preceded binges. Self-monitoring data also confirmed the significance of being alone at work at closing time as an antecedent to binging. These data also suggested that he had difficulty controlling his eating on days that he did not work. Note also that Lanny recorded an average of only 2.64 eating episodes per day. This suggested that this patient was ingesting most of his calories through binging. Thus, treatment planning for eating problems entailed modification of binging at work and at home.

Assessment results for secondary psychopathology showed that Lanny met the diagnostic criteria for dysthymia and avoidant personality disorder. Results from the BISP and BDI suggested significant problems with depression. The BDI score of 24 is suggestive of mild depression. Also, Lanny's MMPI results corroborate this conclusion. An elevation on scale 4 (Pd) suggests problems with impulse control, and elevations on scales 2 (D) and 0 (Si) are typical of socially introverted individuals who have mild but chronic depression. These individuals may lack social skills and may be particularly uncomfortable around members of the opposite sex. His score on the FNE is significantly above the mean, suggesting that he

Table 8.4. Assessment Results

Name: Lanny M.   Client #: B7421

Eating Disorder Measures: Height: 6'1" Weight: 326 BMI: 57

EQ-R: 48 BULIT: 105 EAT: 21

BIA: Current: 9 t = N/A Ideal: 4 t = N/A Difference t-score = N/A

Self-monitoring:

Amount Eaten	#	Hunger		Mood		At Home While Eating (%)	Alone While Eating (%)
		Prior	After	Prior	After		
Undereat	2	4	4	3	3	100	100
Normal	10	3	2	2	2	75	75
Slight Overeat	7	3	2	3	3	85	85
Moderate Overeat	9	5	2	3	4	75	95
Binge	9	4	1	4	5	25	100
Purge	0						

Cal./day = 3250   Eats/day = 2.64   Exercise/day = .25

Secondary Psychopathology:

MMPI Code: 2(t = 78) − 4(t = 75) − 0(t = 69)

Interview Results: Anxiety 6 Depression 16

Comments: dysthymia, avoidant personality features

BDI: 24

FNE: 25

MOCI: Total = 5 Checking = 0 Washing = 0 Slowness = 1 Doubting = 4

FES: (t-scores) Cohesion 59 Expressiveness 45 Conflict 51

Independence 62 Achievement Org. 46 Intellectual-Cultural Org. 47

Active-Recreational 41 Moral-Religious 56 Organization 43 Control 43

greatly feared social rejection and alienation. Further interview inquiry confirmed both the diagnosis of dysthymia and avoidant personality.

Lanny's treatment plan is shown in Table 8.5. While Energy Balance Training was recommended as one component of treatment, additional treatment components were recommended for management of compulsive overeating, dysthymia, and avoidant personality problems. In addition, a relatively new procedure called "Temptation Exposure with Response Prevention" (Johnson, Corrigan, & Mayo, 1987) was recommended. The goal of this procedure is to extinguish urges to binge. The patient is exposed to various binge cues, and then is prevented from engaging in binging. Likely candidates for binge cues for Lanny were the

Table 8.5. Eating Disorder Treatment Plan

Name: _Lanny M._   Age _28_   Sex: _M_

Marital Status: _S_   Occupational Status: _FT, Restaurant Manager_

A. Problem List: 1. _Obesity_

                 2. _Binge eating_

                 3. _Depression_

                 4. _Social anxiety_

B. DSM-III-R Diagnosis:

    Axis 1: 316.00, 307.5: atypical eating disorder, 300.40: dysthymia

    Axis 2: Avoidant personality   Axis 3: Obesity

C. Treatment Plan:

    1. Eating Disorder Therapy: _Decrease binging, decrease_

       calorie intake, EBT: regular meal scheduling, alternative

       responses, TERP: binge foods, alone, boredom, closing at

       work.

    2. Nutrition Therapy: _1500–1800 cal. meal plan_

    3. Other Problems: _Cognitive-behavior therapy for_

       depression, social skills training

sight and smell of his favorite binge foods, being alone, closing at work, and boredom.

Cognitive therapy in combination with social skills training and exposure to social situations were recommended to treat the depression and social isolation. Primary treatment outcome measures for this patient included self-monitoring variables such as number of binges and mood prior to binges. The BDI and the FNE were recommended to systematically evaluate changes in depression and social anxiety.

These two cases illustrate the great diversity of patients who seek treatment for weight loss. Treatment for some patients will be straightforward, relatively short, and quite successful. On the other hand, many obese patients will present with many other problems, such as depression and binge eating. Treatment for these cases is usually much more complicated and longer, with poorer prognosis. Some patients may need to increase their activity (as with June), while others may need to decrease their caloric intake, and most will need to do both. Thus, obese patients exhibit a wide range of problem severity, some with little weight to lose and little other psychopathology; some with a great amount of weight to lose with well-established problem eating behaviors and significant secondary psychopathology. Treatment of more severe cases requires comprehensive evaluation in order to provide clear direction concerning the treatment needed to deal with the specific problem areas.

ANOREXIA NERVOSA

Because of the potential dangers of low weight status and malnutrition, cases of anorexia nervosa must be quickly and carefully evaluated. For most cases, immediate hospitalization will be required. Strong recommendations for inpatient treatment should be made if the patient's weight is below 15 percent underweight, is purging every day, has been resistant to treatment, denies a problem, or has severe secondary psychopathology.

In cases where the eating disorder is denied, information from significant others and direct observation of eating is often essential. After establishing a diagnosis and assessing level of severity, the next focus of assessment should be on core features of anorexia nervosa, such as avoidance of forbidden foods, body image disturbances, and fear of weight gain. Assessment of secondary psychopathology should emphasize marital and/or familial conflict and diagnosis of personality disorders and anxiety or depression. The following case examples illustrate this process.

Case Example. Mary was a college sophomore who was referred to treatment by her family. She weighed 97 lbs. at a height of 5 ft. 3 in. She had lost 20 lbs. in the four months prior to being referred for treatment. In her freshman year of college, Mary had gone to a college in her hometown and had lived at home with her parents. At the time of referral, Mary was living away from home for the first time. She went home almost every weekend however, and had few college friends. Because of her low weight she was hospitalized two weeks after initial presentation. Much of the assessment data were collected during the two weeks prior to hospitalization.

Mary had dated one boyfriend regularly in high school. In her first few months at college she was concerned that she had not received any invitations for dates. While walking to class one day, she passed a group of boys and overheard one saying "yeah, but she has fat thighs." Convinced that he was discussing her, Mary began a very stringent diet with regular exercise (about one hour per day). This exercise gradually increased until at the time of assessment she was exercising two to three hours per day. Mary would let nothing else interfere with her exercise regimen and this resulted in even fewer social contacts. About two weeks after she began the diet and exercise program, she was asked out for her first date while at college. She attributed this invitation to her losing weight and so she implicitly concluded that losing more weight would result in more dates.

Mary's assessment results are summarized in Table 8.6. A relatively low score on the BULIT and self-monitoring data showed that she did not have problems with binging and purging. Her BULIT score was significantly below the cutoff (102) for bulimia, and her self-monitoring showed that she cited a number of "overeats" (that usually involved ingestion of a forbidden food) but no true binging behavior. Note that her self-monitoring shows that she experienced no changes in hunger. This is typical of many anorexics in that they either report no hunger or no significant changes in hunger. Body image assessment indicated that she had serious concerns about her body size. Mary's choice of card 7 on the BIA (t = 83) was more than three standard deviations above the mean for other women her height and weight. Thus, Mary perceived her body size to be

Table 8.6. Assessment Results

Name: _Mary B._____ Client #: _A431249_

Eating Disorder Measures: Height: _5'3"_ Weight: _97 lbs._ BMI: _17.7_

EQ-R: _32_ BULIT: _85_ EAT: _35_

BIA: Current: _7 t = 83_ Ideal: _1 t = 28_ Difference t-score = _55_

Self-monitoring:

		Hunger		Mood		At Home While Eating (%)	Alone While Eating (%)
Amount Eaten	#	Prior	After	Prior	After		
Undereat	11	2	2	3	3	100	100
Normal	4	2	2	2	4	75	85
Slight Overeat	2	2	2	3	5	50	50
Moderate Overeat	1	2	2	3	5	0	0
Binge	0						
Purge	0						

Cal./day = 750   Eats/day = 1.29   Exercise/day = 2.5 hours

Secondary Psychopathology:

MMPI Code: _3(t = 82) − 1(t = 75)_____

Interview Results: Anxiety _8_ Depression _15_

Comments: _some depressive symptoms, possible obsessive features_____

BDI: _19_

MOCI: Total = _16_ Checking = _5_ Washing = _2_ Slowness = _5_ Doubting = _4_

FES: (t-scores) Cohesion _62_ Expressiveness _48_ Conflict _53_

Independence _44_ Achievement Org. _55_ Intellectual-Cultural Org. _55_

Active _56_ Moral-Religious _48_ Organization _60_ Control _60_ much larger than normal. Mary's choice of card 1 (t = 28) for her ideal body size was significantly below the mean for her body size. Not only did she perceive herself to be "fat," but she wanted to be thinner than most women her size. Therefore, Mary had significant body image distortion (as indicated by the high current BIA score), she also strongly preferred a thin body size (as suggested by the low ideal BIA score), and consequently expressed severe dissatisfaction with body size (as indicated by the large difference between the two BIA scores). Gradual increase in caloric intake, treatment of body concerns, restructuring of irrational beliefs regarding weight loss, and some attention to anxiety and depression issues were recommended in this case. Table 8.7 summarizes the diagnosis and treatment plan for Mary. Critical components of her treatment in addition to hospitalization included Energy Balance Training and treatment of body image concerns. In addition, we established a plan to help her modify dysfunctional beliefs regarding weight loss and her fear of fat.

With regard to secondary psychopathology, Mary had elevations on MMPI scales 1 (Hs) and 3 (Hy) which suggested histrionic characteristics. Mary's roommate was involved in treatment so that she could learn to

Table 8.7. Eating Disorder Treatment Plan

Name: Mary B. _____ Age _20_ Sex: _F_

Marital Status: _S_ Occupational Status: _FT Student_____

A. Problem List: 1. _Restrictive eating_____
                  2. _Body image concerns_____
                  3. _Fear of "fatness"_____
                  4. _Dysfunctional weight loss beliefs_____
                  5. _Histrionic features_____
                  6. _Obsessive-compulsive behaviors_____

B. DSM-III-R Diagnosis:
   Axis 1: 307.10: anorexia nervosa
   Axis 2: histrionic traits   Axis 3: None

C. Treatment Plan:
   1. Eating Disorder Therapy: _Immediate hospitalization,_____
      _increase calorie intake, Energy Balance Training,_____
      cognitive restructuring re: weight loss beliefs, fear of
      _fat. Body image treatment._____
   2. Nutrition Therapy: _Increase calorie intake gradually,____
      _proper nutrition training._____
   3. Other Problems: _Exposure with Response Prevention regarding_
      _obsessive-compulsive checking and ordering._____

avoid providing excessive attention for Mary's dysfunctional eating habits. Thus, her roommate was instructed to praise Mary when she ate normal meals but to try and ignore her when she restricted her eating or began complaining about "how fat" she was. Finally, results from the Maudsley Obsessive-Compulsive Inventory (MOCI) led to further investigation of obsessive-compulsive disorder. Her total score (16) was close to that observed in obsessionals (Hodgson & Rachman, 1977) and was more than two standard deviations above that of normals (Dent & Slakovskis, 1986). Her scores on the slowness and the checking subscales of the MOCI were well above the mean. Further inquiry showed that obsessive-compulsive checking related to safety and orderliness interfered with her social functioning. Exposure with response prevention and administration of the antidepressant medication, Prozac, was recommended. Treatment outcome was evaluated using self-monitoring procedures to measure number of normal eating episodes, calorie intake, and the types of foods that were eaten. Evaluation of obsessive-compulsive checking and ordering was evaluated using the MOCI and direct observation of these behaviors during exposure treatment sessions.

Case Example. Debra was an anorexic patient who engaged in purgative behavior as well as restrictive eating. At the time of assessment, Debra had been divorced for ten years, lived with her sister, and her romantic partner had recently ended their relationship. Also, it was evident from the interview that Debra was relatively alienated from her family. Debra reported that she had "always been on a diet," but since this breakup a month and a half before assessment, she lost 15 lbs. and weighed 91 lbs. at 5 ft. 3 in. Thus her BMI was 16.8, below the suggested cutoff for anorexia. Table 8.8 summarizes her assessment results.

Both of Debra's parents were extremely obese. When she was young, other children reportedly teased her because of her parents' obesity. Shortly after puberty, Debra gained 15 lbs. in two months. One may observe that at this point Debra was at step three, the "fatness" stage of the etiological model described in Chapter 1 (Figure 1.2). This is the stage where the individual has a subjective experience of being overweight. This weight gain "scared" Debra and she immediately went on a diet. She reported that she had tried many restrictive diets since this time. When she was 17 she began purging. Debra had been on a very restrictive diet for two months when she read an article in a woman's magazine about bulimia. After trying to purge once and swearing that she would "never do that again," several weeks later she induced vomiting again and recalled that it was easier this time. Slowly this purgative behavior became more frequent, but Debra never really developed the binging typical of bulimia nervosa.

Table 8.8. Assessment Results

Name: __Debra W.__   Client #: __A39047__

Eating Disorder Measures: Height: __5'5"__   Weight: __91 lbs.__   BMI: __16.8__

EQ-R: __35__   BULIT: __115__   EAT: __69__

BIA: Current: __4 t = 59__   Ideal: __1 t = 28__   Difference t-score = __31__

Self-monitoring:
No self-monitoring data available due to hospitalization.

Secondary Psychopathology:
MMPI Code: __Scale 4(t = 85) − 2(t = 79) − 8(t = 74)__

Interview Results: Anxiety __9__   Depression __19__

Comments: __major depression, characteristics of borderline__
__personality disorder__

BDI: __35__

FNE: __121__

MOCI: Total = __9__ Checking = __3__ Washing = __2__ Slowness = __1__ Doubting = __3__

FES: (t-scores) Cohesion __22__   Expressiveness __24__   Conflict __75__

Independence __44__   Achievement Org. __41__   Intellectual-Cultural Org. __40__

Active __46__   Moral-Religious __55__   Organization __46__   Control __80__

Comments: __patient was resistant to assessment procedure, is very__
__unhappy about being in the hospital.__

Scores on the EAT (>40) and self-monitoring data indicated that Debra was a restrictive eater. At the time of referral Debra purged most of the food she ate. This bulimic behavior was reflected by elevated BULIT (>102) and EQ-R scores. Because of her very low weight and frequent purging, Debra was hospitalized immediately. Her treatment plan is summarized in Table 8.9. In the hospital, initial treatment focused on eating behavior. Initially a meal plan of 1200 calories was prescribed, and both her eating behavior at meals and her postmeal behavior (to prevent purging) were carefully monitored. In the following weeks, her caloric intake was gradually increased. We find that comprehensive inpatient treatment for patients such as Debra often takes six weeks and many times is even longer. Thus, both the patient and her friends and family should be prepared for a lengthy stay in the hospital.

Debra's results on the MMPI showed elevations on scales 4 (Pd), 2 (D), and 8 (Sc). This pattern suggested that she had characteristics of borderline personality disorder. Thus, clear limits were established with the client, and the staff was warned to recognize staff splitting (attempting to turn the staff against each other). Also the potential for Debra to sabotage treatment or engage in self-injurious behavior was noted. The patient

Table 8.9. Eating Disorder Treatment Plan

Name: _Debra W._____ Age _32_ Sex: _F_
Marital Status: _S_ Occupational Status: _FT Secretary_____
A. Problem List: 1. _Restrictive eating_____
              2. _Purging_____
              3. _Fear of "fatness"_____
              4. _Borderline behaviors_____

B. DSM-III-R Diagnosis:
    Axis 1: 307.1: anorexia nervosa, 297.22: major depression
    Axis 2: 301.83: borderline P.D.   Axis 3: Deferred

C. Treatment Plan:
    1. Eating Disorder Therapy: _Immediate hospitalization,_____
       increase calorie intake, prevent purging, cognitive_____
       restructuring re: "fear of fatness"_____

    2. Nutrition Therapy: _Gradually increase calorie intake____
       from 1200 calories, proper nutrition counseling_____
    3. Other Problems: _Cognitive-behavior treatment of_____
       depression, consider antidepressant medication, family_____
       therapy to improve communication and conflict, and_____
       increase family cohesion to help provide stronger social_____
       support for patient_____

attempted to turn the staff against each other in her first few weeks of treatment. However, because the hospital staff was alerted to this possibility it did not significantly interfere with treatment. Her score on the BDI is in the severe depression range, which is also typical of some borderline patients. Therefore antidepressant medication was recommended for this patient.

Debra's alienation from her family was indicated in the results obtained from the FES. The data suggested that her family was low in cohesion, tolerated little emotional expression by family members, and also had frequent conflict. Thus a recommendation was made for family therapy as well.

In addition to weight increases as measured by the BMI, other important outcome measures for this patient were the BULIT, EAT, and EQ-R. Also, observation of the eating of forbidden foods when in the hospital were noted. Upon hospital discharge, Debra's self-monitoring data was an important indicator of the success of treatment and the maintenance of treatment gains. Particular self-monitoring variables that we felt were important were number of undereats, number of normal eats, mood and hunger prior to and after undereats, and finally the eating of forbidden foods.

These two patients illustrate different treatment protocols that may be required when dealing with anorexic patients. While anorexic individuals may be treated on an outpatient basis, most anorexics will require hospitalization for treatment to be successful. These cases also point out the importance of evaluating the presence of excessive exercise and/or purging behavior. Finally, the clinician should be prepared for a relatively long and sometimes frustrating treatment process with these patients. Treatment recommendations may have to be changed more than once, and several different intervention techniques may be required. Thus, with these patients the assessment process must continue throughout treatment so that treatment planning may be readily changed when needed.

BULIMIA NERVOSA

As a group, bulimics tend to be somewhat less resistant than anorexics. Usually the younger the patient, the more likely resistance. Most bulimics respond well to group therapy for eating problems and need no other intervention, but some require individual therapy in addition to group treatment. Bulimics who require inpatient treatment are generally those characterized by frequent binging and purging, significant levels of depression, and severe personality disturbances such as borderline personality. Also, we find that hospitalization is required when the bulimic has been in outpatient treatment for a significant amount of time but has not responded as expected. The following case examples illustrate how these treatment decisions can be made based on assessment data.

Case Example. Jackie was a 21-year-old senior in college seeking treatment for bulimia nervosa. At the time of assessment Jackie was living with her family. She was of normal weight (124 lbs., 5 ft. 4 in.) but wanted to lose at least 10 lbs. She had a steady boyfriend, who insisted that she seek treatment. In interview, it was revealed that Jackie felt that her father never loved her. Jackie's mother sensed this perceived rejection of Jackie by her father, and so was especially nurturing to Jackie. Reportedly, this caused Jackie and her mother to be very close, while Jackie's father was more distanced from the family. One may note the low cohesion and higher conflict scores from Jackie's FES in Table 8.10. In addition, low independence and high religiosity scores were reflective of the strict family rules that were placed on Jackie. She also recalled how her father would point out the women on television with attractive figures. Thus, Jackie implicitly concluded that she could get her father's attention and respect by having an attractive figure.

Table 8.10. Assessment Results

Name: Jackie P. _____ Client #: B8769

Eating Disorder Measures: Height: 5'4" Weight: 124 lbs. BMI: 22

EQ-R: 43 BULIT: 118 EAT: 42

BIA: Current: 7 t = 69 Ideal: 2 t = 35 Difference t-score = 34

Self-monitoring: Cal./day = 1875

		Hunger		Mood		At Home While Eating (%)	Alone While Eating (%)
Amount Eaten	#	Prior	After	Prior	After		
Undereat	2	2	2	3	3	85	45
Normal	7	3	1	3	4	75	50
Slight Overeat	0						
Moderate Overeat	3	4	1	3	4	33	33
Binge	10	5	1	5	5	100	100
Purge	10	1	3	5	5	100	100

Purging after binges = 100% Purging after nonbinges = 0%

Secondary Psychopathology:

MMPI Code: 4(t = 75) − 2(t = 71) − 0(t = 69) _____

Interview Results: Anxiety 6 Depression 10

Comments: some depressive symptoms, very sensitive to social feedback

BDI: 18

FNE: 28

MOCI: Total = 6 Checking = 0 Washing = 0 Slowness = 1 Doubting = 5

FES: (t-scores)Cohesion 28 Expressiveness 40 Conflict 69

Independence 22 Achievement Org. 51 Intellectual-Cultural Org. 81

Active 46 Moral-Religious 77 Organization 59 Control 75

When Jackie was 16 and was no more than 5 lbs. overweight, she went on a fast and lost 15 lbs. in about one month. When eligible dates commented on her weight loss, Jackie concluded that she had found the solution to getting attention from boys. Thus she proceeded to attempt various restrictive diets. However, she found that after a few weeks on these diets, she "could never hold out" and she would then binge on foods such as pastries and candy-coated chocolates. This binging was always done in secrecy. During the period of restrictive dieting and occasional binging, she found that she could no longer lose weight, and instead gained a few pounds. This weight gain was quite distressing and eventually she attempted self-induced vomiting. Her purgative behavior gradually increased in frequency. This behavior continued until the time of referral. She reported that her binging and purging was often exacerbated by disruptions in the home. The impact of stress from the home is also supported by her self-monitoring data. As seen in Table 8.10, her binges were invariably at home, and many times they followed family conflict.

Jackie's assessment results are summarized in Table 8.10. These data are typical of many bulimic patients. It was evident from self-monitoring and from the interview that Jackie's purging (via self-induced vomiting) was directly related to her binging. Note from Table 8.10 that her purges always follow a binge (100%). Table 8.11 describes this patient's treatment plan. The first treatment goal was elimination of purging using Exposure with Response Prevention (ERP). Briefly, this procedure entails exposing the patient to the consumption of typical binge foods with prevention of purgative habits. The effect of this procedure is to reduce the anxiety associated with eating certain feared foods.

When purging was reduced, Jackie began to restrict her eating. After one and a half months of treatment with exposure plus response prevention, self-monitoring data showed that she had virtually ceased purging, but she was now avoiding many foods and her caloric intake had decreased significantly. Also, she was losing weight. Table 8.12 provides Jackie's assessment results following two months of treatment. It was apparent that she was avoiding forbidden foods. After two additional

Table 8.11. Eating Disorder Treatment Plan

Name: Jackie P.   Age 23   Sex: F

Marital Status: S   Occupational Status: FT student

A. Problem List: 1. Binging
2. Purging
3. Body image concerns
4. Social anxiety (interpersonal sensitivity)
5. Family problems

B. DSM-III-R Diagnosis:
Axis 1: 307.51: bulimia nervosa
Axis 2: 301.82: avoidant P.D.   Axis 3: None

C. Treatment Plan:
1. Eating Disorder Therapy: Decrease purging using Exposure with Response Prevention, body image therapy
2. Nutrition Therapy: 1600–2000 calorie meal plan

3. Other Problems: Social skills training, family therapy

Table 8.12. Eating Disorder Treatment Progress

Name: Jackie P.

Date: (2 mos. in treatment)   Weight: 125   BUILT: 97   EAT: 49   BDI: 16

Eating Disorder: Jackie has not purged now for three weeks.
However, her self-monitoring data now indicate that she is avoiding
food (650 ca./day), particularly her forbidden foods. This
behavior was also observed in the ERP session.

Other Problems: J. reports enjoying the group more and
participates more frequently. She also reports more social
activities this week with less anxiety.

weeks of outpatient treatment was unsuccessful in increasing her consumption of forbidden foods or caloric intake, we elected to recommend
hospitalization for this patient. In the hospital, the first step in treatment
was to systematically introduce the consumption of the foods which she
most feared, in addition to establishing and monitoring a regular meal
schedule.

The FES suggested that her family was characterized by low cohesion,
low independence, high intellectual-cultural orientation, high moral-religious orientation, and high control. Subsequent interviews with both
Jackie and other family members determined that family conflict often set
the occasion for binging and purging. Thus, involvment of the family in
treatment was recommended. In family therapy, we focused on education
of how family conflict contributed to Jackie's eating problems and encouraged alternate means of resolving conflict. For example, role playing of
compromise and an egalitarian approach to conflict resolution was a main
component of family therapy.

Jackie's responses on the MMPI and the FNE suggested that she was
avoidant of social interactions and overly sensitive to social rejection.
Treatment was directed toward expanding her social contacts and dealing
with her social sensitivity.

Clients such as these often resist becoming involved with group treatment because they are uncomfortable being in the group. However,
involvement in the group can often help desensitize this social anxiety.
Thus, changes in the FNE score were targeted as an important treatment
outcome measure. In addition, scores from the BULIT, EAT, and EQ-R
were chosen for treatment evaluation. Reduction in binging and purging
were also selected as primary variables for evaluating changes in bulimia.

Case Example. Maxine was a 29-year-old patient referred for treatment
at the encouragement of her husband. Although Maxine binged occasion-

ally (about three times per week), she was best characterized as a restric-tive eater. She did not purge through self-induced vomiting or laxative abuse. However, from information gained through interview and self-monitoring it was found that exercise served as a purgative habit. If dietary restraint was violated, Maxine always went to the exercise club to work out for at least two hours. Such clients usually do not recognize this type of exercise as a purgative habit and may resist this suggestion for some time in treatment. Table 8.13 summarizes the results of assessment and Table 8.14 summarizes the recommended treatment plan. Exposure with Response Prevention was recommended in this case. Here, the behavior prevented following eating was exercise. We also suggested a healthier exercise program which did not follow meals, gradually

Table 8.13. Assessment Results

Name: _Maxine_____ Client #: _B0187_

Eating Disorder Measures: Height: _5'6"_ Weight: _119 lbs._ BMI: _19.2_

EQ-R: _45_ BULIT: _105_ EAT: _65_

BIA: Current: _6 t = 66_ Ideal: _2 t = 37_ Difference t-score = _29_

Self-monitoring: Cal./day = 650 Exercise/day = 2.5 hrs.

Amount Eaten	#	Hunger		Mood		At Home While Eating (%)	Alone While Eating (%)
		Prior	After	Prior	After		
Undereat	7	3	3	3	3	100	57
Normal	7	3	2	2	3	86	86
Slight Overeat	7	4	2	3	3	100	86
Moderate Overeat	6	5	2	3	3	80	80
Binge	1	5	1	2	3	100	100
Purge	0						

Eats/day = 2.0 Exercise/day = 2.5 hrs.

Comments: _Exercise serves as functional purge. Also, her cal._
intake on days when she has a significant dispute with her husband
declines to 350 cal.

Secondary Psychopathology:

MMPI Code: _3(t = 82) − 4(t = 75) − 6(t = 72), low 5 (t = 31)_

Interview Results: Anxiety _7_ Depression _10_ BDI: _16_

MOCI: Total = _7_ Checking = _4_ Washing = _0_ Slowness = _1_ Doubting = _2_

FES: (t-scores) Cohesion _45_ Expressiveness _45_ Conflict _65_

Independence _52_ Achievement Org. _45_ Intellectual-Cultural Org. _43_

Active _59_ Moral-Religious _43_ Organization _52_ Control _57_

DAS: 83, spouse = 93

Table 8.14. Eating Disorder Treatment Plan

Name: _Maxine S._ _____ Age _29_ Sex: _F_

Marital Status: _M_ Occupational Status: _PT sales_____

A. Problem List: 1. _Restrictive eating_____
              2. _Extensive exercise_____
              3. _Purging through exercise_____
              4. _Excessive body concern_____
              5. _Passive-aggressive behaviors_____
              6. Marital discord_____

B. DSM-III-R Diagnosis:
   Axis 1: 307.51:bulimia nervosa
   Axis 2: 301.84: passive-aggressive Axis 3: None

C. Treatment Plan:
   1. Eating Disorder Therapy: _Energy Balance Training,_____
      increase calories, body image treatment, Exposure with
      Response Prevention, decrease exercise following meals
   2. Nutrition Therapy: Therapy: _Increase caloric intake_____
   3. Other Problems: _Assertiveness training, marital therapy_____

increased caloric intake, and treatment of her body image and fear of weight gain.

Because this patient reported significant marital discord during the BISP, she and her spouse were administered the Dyadic Adjustment Scale (DAS). The results from the DAS revealed significant marital dissatisfaction for both Maxine and her partner. Maxine's DAS score was significantly below the 100 cutoff indicating marital satisfaction. While her spouse also scored below this cutoff, his score was higher indicating more marital satisfaction. Thus, as with many bulimics who are married, Maxine was more dissatisfied with her marriage than was her partner (Van Buren & Williamson, 1988). The results of self-monitoring showed that there was a close relationship between marital arguments and caloric intake. The more arguments they had, the fewer calories Maxine would consume. Maxine's MMPI profile suggested passive-aggressive tendencies (high scale 4-Pd, low scale 5-Mf, high scale 6-Pa). In this case, mood appeared to have a less direct relationship to her eating behavior than did problems with her husband. Observation of self-monitoring data in Table 8.13 shows no obvious relationship between mood and restricting or overeating. We felt that it would be best to include Maxine's husband in treatment and also referred them for marital therapy.

For the evaluation of effectiveness of treatment, the BULIT, EAT, and EQ-R were deemed most appropriate. Also, self-monitoring of eating and

exercise behavior was carefully evaluated. Finally, body image disturbances were monitored via the BIA.

These two bulimia cases illustrate how a similar underlying problem
(fear of weight gain) may result in two quite different modes of purging,
self-induced vomiting for Jackie, and exercise for Maxine. Also, these
examples emphasize the importance of continuing assessment. For Jackie,
this led to hospitalization and, for Maxine, ongoing assessment identified
the need for marital therapy. Finally, these cases highlight the importance
of the assessment of family variables when planning treatment.

Summary

The examples in this chapter described how assessment procedures can
be used for developing individual treatment plans. The case examples
were presented to illustrate the great diversity among eating disorder
patients. Even though patients may carry the same eating disorder diagnosis, they may require distinctly different treatment protocols. Each client, no matter how similar, may be experiencing a unique set of stressors
that may interact with the eating disorder. As the cases in this chapter
illustrate, life stressors often exacerbate eating problems and must be considered when developing a treatment plan.

The ideosyncratic nature of each eating disorder patient also brings out
the importance of a thorough assessment of secondary psychopathology.
As depicted in the case examples, secondary psychopathology often has
important implications for treatment planning. Personality problems such
as interpersonal sensitivity and borderline personality disorder may interfere with treatment by leading to avoidance of group therapy or staff splitting. Treatment planning that does not adequately consider the impact of
personality variables on the process of treatment will likely be
unsuccessful.

There are several assessment issues that become important for all eating disorder diagnoses. The extent of overweight or underweight status
of a client will determine both the immediacy and the direction of treatment. Seriously underweight patients will probably need inpatient treatment, while severely overweight individuals will require long-term outpatient treatment for weight loss. Self-monitoring data are essential not
just for initial evaluations, but for the ongoing evaluation of treatment as
well. In addition, the presence of binge eating should be investigated for
all eating disorder patients. Specific treatment planning for binging is
essential if it is determined that this is a problem eating behavior. We
should also emphasize the value of nutritional counseling for virtually all
eating disorder clients. Whether the nutritional counseling seeks to assist

the obese patient in making wise food choices, or seeks to correct the misbeliefs regarding both food and weight gain that is typical in anorexia and bulimia, this is a valuable facet of treatment for eating disorder clients.

One of the important questions that will confront the clinician in the assessment of eating disorders is the question of hospitalization. Several issues relate to whether the clinician decides that inpatient treatment is in the best interests of the client. Weight status, extent of the problem eating behaviors, extent of secondary psychopathology, and the success of ongoing outpatient treatment are all considerations which may assist the clinician in making this determination.

Finally, it should be emphasized that the assessment process never really ends. It is often the case that we are well into treatment before the full spectrum of the client's problems becomes evident. Also, it is important for the clinician to keep abreast of the ongoing progress (or regression) of the eating disorder patient while in treatment. Thus, as with all science, it is good for the clinician to always keep the patient's formulation tentative, with the full realization that conceptualization of the problem, and the treatment, may require revision during the process of treatment.

References

Agras, W. S. (1987). *Eating disorders: Management of obesity, bulimia, and anorexia nervosa.* New York: Pergamon Press.

Allebeck, P., Hallberg, D., & Espmark, S. (1976). Body image: An apparatus for measuring disturbances in estimation of size and shape. *Journal of Psychosomatic Research, 20,* 583–589.

American Psychiatric Association. (1980). *Diagnostic and statistical manual of mental disorders* (3rd ed.). Washington: Author.

American Psychiatric Association. (1987). *Diagnostic and statistical manual of mental disorders* (3rd ed.-rev.). Washington: Author.

Apfelbaum, M. (1975). Influence of level of energy intake in man: Effects of spontaneous intake on experimental starvation and experimental overeating. In G. A. Bray (Ed.), *Obesity in Perspective* (pp. 27–30). Washington, DC: U.S. Government Printing Office.

Apfelbaum, M., Bostsarron, J., & Lacatis, D. (1971). Effect of caloric restriction and excessive caloric intake on energy expenditure. *American Journal of Clinical Nutrition, 24,* 1405–1409.

Beck, A. T. & Beamesderfer, A. (1974). Assessment of depression: The depression inventory. In P. Pichot (Ed.), *Psychological measurements in phsychopharmacology: Moden problems in pharmapsychiatry, Vol. 7.* Paris: Karger, Basil.

Bellack, A. S. & Williamson, D. A. (1980). Obesity and anorexia nervosa. In Doleys, D. M., Meredith, R. L., & Ciminero, A. R. (Eds.), *Behavioral Psychology in Medicine: Assessment and Treatment Strategies,* (pp. 295–316). New York: Plenum Publishing Corp.

Bennett, S. M., Williamson, D. A., & Powers, S. K. (1989). Bulimia nervosa and resting metabolic rate. *International Journal of Eating Disorders, 8,* 417–424.

Ben-Tovim, D. I. & Crisp, A. H. (1984). The reliability of estimates of body width and their relationship to current measured body size among anorexic and normal subjects. *Psychological Medicine, 14,* 843–846.

Berscheid, E., Walster, E., & Bohrnstedt, G. (1973, November). The happy American body: A survey report. *Psychology Today,* pp. 119–131.

Beumont, P., Al-Alami, M., & Touyz, S. (1988). Relevance of a standard measurement of undernutrition to the diagnosis of anorexia nervosa: Use of Quetelet's body mass index (BMI). *International Journal of Eating Disorders, 7,* 399–405.

Billewicz, W. Z., Kemsley, W. F. F., & Thomson A. M. (1962). Indices of adiposity. *British Journal of Preventive Social Medicine, 16,* 183–188.

Birtchnell, S. A., Lacey, J. H., & Harte, A. (1985). Body image distortion in bulimia nervosa. *British Journal of Psychiatry, 147,* 408–412.

Bjorntorp, P. (1977). The fat cell: A clinical review. In G. A. Bray (Ed.), *Recent Advances in Obesity Research: II* (pp. 153–168). Los Angeles: Newman Publishing.

Bjorntorp, P., Karlsson, M., Gustafsson, L., Smith, U., Sjostrom, L., Cigolini, M., Storck, G., & Pettersson, P. (1979). Quantitation of different cells in the epididymal fat pad of the rat. *Journal of Lipid Research, 20,* 97–106.

Bloom, W. L. & Eidex, M. F. (1967). Inactivity as a major factor in adult obesity. *Metabolism, 16,* 679–684.

Brantley, P. J., Cocke, T. B., Jones, G. N., & Goreczny, A. J. (1988). The Daily Stress Inventory: Validity and effect of repeated administration. *Journal of Psychopathology and Behavioral Assessment, 10,* 75–81.

Brantley, P. J., Waggoner, C. D., Jones, G. N., & Rappaport, N. B. (1987). A Daily Stress Inventory: Development, reliability, and validity. *Journal of Behavioral Medicine, 10,* 61–74.

Brownell, K. D. & Stunkard, A.J. (1980). Physical activity in the development and control of obesity. In A. J. Stunkard (Ed.), *Obesity* (pp. 300–324). Philadelphia: W. B. Saunders Co.

Bruch, H. (1973). *Eating disorders: Anorexia nervosa, obesity and the person within.* New York: Basic Books.

Bulik, C. M. (1987). Drug and alcohol abuse by bulimic women and their families. *American Journal of Psychiatry, 144,* 1604–1606.

Button, E. J., Fransella, F., & Slade, P. D. (1977). A reappraisal of body perception disturbance in anorexia nervosa. *Psychological Medicine, 7,* 235–243.

Carlson, G. A. & Cantwell, P. P. (1980). Unmasking masked depression in children and adolescents. *American Journal of Psychiatry, 37,* 445–449.

Cash, T. F. & Brown, T. A. (1987). Body image in anorexia nervosa and bulimia nervosa: A review of the literature. *Behavior Modification, 11,* 487–521.

Casper, R. C., Halmi, K. A., Goldberg, S. C., Eckert, E. D., & Davis, J. M. (1979). Disturbances in body image estimation as related to other characteristics and outcome in anorexia nervosa. *British Journal of Psychiatry, 134,* 60–66.

Chirico, A. M. & Stunkard, A. J. (1960). Physical activity and human obesity. *New England Journal of Medicine, 263,* 935–940.

Choca, J. P., Peterson, C. A., & Shanley, L. A. (1986). Factor analysis of the Millon Clinical Multiaxial Inventory. *Journal of Consulting and Clinical Psychology, 54,* 253–255.

Cooper, Z. & Fairburn, C. G. (1987). The eating disorder examination: A semi-structured interview for the assessment of the specific psychopathology of eating disorders. *International Journal of Eating Disorders, 6,* 1–8.

Counts, C. R. & Adams, H. E. (1985). Body image in bulimic, dieting, and normal females. *Journal of Psychopathology and Behavioral Assessment, 7,* 289–301.

Crisp, A. H. (1970). Premorbid factors in adult disorders of weight, with particular reference to primary anorexia nervosa (weight phobia). A literature review. *Journal of Psychosomatic Research, 14,* 1–22.

Crisp, A. H. & Kalucy, R. S. (1974). Aspects of the perceptual disorder in anorexia nervosa. *British Journal of Medical Psychology, 47,* 349–361.

Cronk, C. E. & Roche, A. F. (1982). Race- and sex-specific reference data for triceps and subscapular skinfolds and weight/stature. *The American Journal of Clincial Nutrition, 35,* 347–354.

Dally, P. J. (1969). *Anorexia nervosa.* New York: Grune & Stratton.

Davis, C. J., Williamson, D. A., Goreczny, A. J., & Bennett, S. M. (1989). Body image disturbances and bulimia nervosa: An empirical analysis of recent revisions of DSM-III. *Journal of Psychopathology and Behavioral Assessment, 11,* 61–69.

Davis, R., Freeman, R. J., & Garner, D. M. (1988). A naturalistic investigation of eating behavior in bulimia nervosa. *Journal of Consulting and Clinical Psychology, 56,* 273–279.

DeLongis, A., Coyne, J. C., Dakof, G., Folkman, S., & Lazarus, R. S. (1982). Relationship of daily hassles, uplifts, and major life events to health status. *Health Psychology, 1,* 119–136.

Dent, H. R. & Slakovskis, P. M. (1986). Clinical measures of depression, anxiety and obsessionality in non-clinical populations. *Behaviour Research and Therapy, 24,* 689–691.

Derogatis, L. R. (1977). *SCL-90 administration, scoring and procedures manual-I.* Baltimore: Johns Hopkins University Press.

DiNardo, S. A., O'Brien, G. T., Barlow, D. H., Waddell, M. T., & Blanchard, E. B. (1983). Reliability of DSM-III anxiety categories using a new structured interview. *Archives of General Psychiatry, 40,* 1070–1075.

Duchmann, E. G., Williamson, D. A., & Stricker, P. M. (1989). Bulimia, dietary restraint, and concern for dieting. *Journal of Psychopathology and Behavioral Assessment, 11,* 1–13.

Durnin, J. V. G. A. & Womersley, J. (1974). Body fat assessed from total body density and its estimation from skinfold thickness: Measurements on 481 men and women aged from 16 to 72 years. *British Journal of Psychiatry, 32,* 32–77.

Edwin, D., Andersen, A. E., & Rosell, F. (1988). Outcome prediction by MMPI subtypes of anorexia nervosa. *Psychosomatic Medicine, 29,* 273–282.

Endicott, J. & Spitzer, R. L. (1978). A diagnostic interview: The schedule for affective disorders and schizophrenia. *Archives of General Psychiatry, 15,* 249–255.

Fairburn, C. G. & Cooper, P. J. (1982). Self-induced vomiting and bulimia nervosa: An undetected problem. *British Medical Journal, 284,* 1153–1155.

Fairburn, C. G. & Garner, D. M. (1986). The diagnosis of bulimia nervosa. *International Journal of Eating Disorders, 5,* 403–419.

Farquharson, R. F. & Hyland, H. H. (1966). Anorexia nervosa: The course of 15 patients treated from 20 to 30 years previously. *Canadian Medical Association Journal, 94,* 411–419.

Fisher, S. & Cleveland, S. E. (1958). *Body image and personality.* New York: Dover.

Foch, T. T. & McClearn, G. E. (1980). Genetics, body weight, and obesity. In A. J. Stunkard (Ed.), *Obesity* (pp. 48–71). Philadelphia: W. B. Saunders.

Foreyt, J. P. (1987). Issues in the assessment and treatment of obesity. *Journal of Consulting and Clinical Psychology, 55,* 677–684.

Freeman, R. J., Thomas, C. D., Solyom, L., & Hunter, M. A. (1984). A modified video camera for measuring body image distortion: Technical description and reliability. *Psychological Medicine, 14,* 411–416.

Freeman, R. J., Thomas, C. D., Solyom, L., & Koopman, R. F. (1985). Clinical and personality correlates of body size overestimation in anorexia nervosa and bulimia nervosa. *International Journal of Eating Disorders, 4,* 439–456.

Freeman, R. J., Thomas, C. D., Solyom, L., & Miles, J. E. (1983). Body image disturbances in anorexia nervosa: A reexamination and a new technique. In P. L. Darby, P. E. Garfinkel, D. M. Garner, & D. V. Coscina (Eds.), *Anorexia nervosa: Recent developments in research* (pp. 117–127). New York: Alan R. Liss.

Garfinkel, P. E., Kaplan, A. S., Garner, D. M., & Darby, P. L. (1983). The differentiation of vomiting and weight loss as a conversion disorder from anorexia nervosa. *American Journal of Psychiatry, 140,* 1019–1022.

Garfinkel, P. E., Moldofsky, H., & Garner, D. M. (1979). The stability of perceptual disturbance in anorexia nervosa. *Psychological Medicine, 9,* 703–708.

Garfinkel, P. E., Moldofsky, H., Garner, D. M., Stancer, H. C., & Coscina, D. V. (1978). Disturbances in "body image" and "satiety." *Psychosomatic Medicine, 40,* 487–498.

Garner, D. M. & Garfinkel, P. E. (1979). The eating attitudes test: An index of the symptoms of anorexia nervosa. *Psychological Medicine, 9,* 273–279.

Garner, D. M. & Garfinkel, P. E. (1981). Body image in anorexia nervosa: Measurement, theory, and clinical implications. *International Journal of Psychiatry in Medicine, 11,* 263–284.

Garner, D. M. Garfinkel, P. E., Schwartz, D., & Thompson, M. (1980). Cultural expectations of thinness in women. *Psychological Reports, 47,* 483–491.

Garner, D. M. & Olmstead, M. P. (1984). *Manual for the Eating Attitudes Test (EDI).* Odessa, FL: Psychological Assessment Resources, Inc.

Garner, D. M., Olmstead, M. P., & Polivy, J. (1983). Development and validation of a multidimensional eating disorder inventory for anorexia nervosa and bulimia. *International Journal of Eating Disorders, 2,* 15–34.

Garner, D. M., Olmstead, M. P. Polivy, J., & Garfinkel, P. E. (1983). Comparison between weight-preoccupied women and anorexia nervosa. *Psychosomatic Medicine, 46,* 255–266.

Garrow, J. S. (1983). Indices of adiposity. *Reviews in Clinical Nutrition, 53,* 697–708.

Garrow, J. S. (1986). Physiological aspects of obesity. In K. D. Brownell & J. P. Foreyt (Eds.), *Handbook of eating disorders: Physiology, psychology, and treatment of obesity, anorexia, and bulimia* (pp. 45–62). New York: Basic Books, Inc.

Gilbertini, M. & Retzlaff, P. D. (1988). Factor invariance of the Millon Clinical Multiaxial Inventory. *Journal of Psychopathology and Behavioral Assessment, 10,* 65–74.

Giles, T. R., Young, R. R. & Young, D. E. (1985). Behavioral treatment of severe bulimia. *Behavior Therapy, 16,* 393–405.

Glucksman, M. L. & Hirsch, J. (1969). The response of obese patients to weight reduction: III. The perceptions of body size. *Psychosomatic Medicine, 31,* 1–7.

Gomez, J. & Dally, P. (1980). Psychometric rating in the assessment of progress in anorexia nervosa. *British Journal of Psychiatry, 136,* 290–296.

Gottesman, E. G. & Caldwell, W. E. (1966). The body-image identification test: A quantitative projective technique to study an aspect of body image. *Journal of Genetic Psychology, 108,* 19–33.

Gross, J., Rosen, J. C., Leitenberg, H., & Willmuth, M. (1986). Validity of Eating Attitudes Test and the Eating Disorders Inventory in bulimia nervosa. *Journal of Consulting and Clinical Psychology, 54,* 875–876.

Gull, N. W. (1874). Anorexia nervosa (apepsia hysterica, anorexia hysterica). *Transactions of Clinical Endocrinological Metabolism, 49,* 806–809.

Halmi, A. C. (1974). Anorexia nervosa: Demographic and clinical features. *Psychosomatic Medicine, 36,* 18–25.

Hamilton, E. W. & Abramson, L. Y. (1983). Cognitive pattern of major depressive disorder: A longitudinal study in a hospital setting. *Journal of Abnormal Psychology, 92,* 174–184.

Hamilton, M. (1959). The assessment of anxiety states by rating. *British Journal of Medical Psychology, 32,* 56–62.

Hamilton, M. (1960). A rating scale for depression. *Journal of Neurology, Neurosurgery, and Psychiatry, 23,* 56–61.

Hamilton, M. (1967). Development of a rating scale for primary depressive illness. *British Journal of School and Clinical Psychology, 6,* 278–296.

Hathaway, S. & McKinley, J. (1951). *MMPI manual, revised edition.* New York: The Psychological Corporation.

Head, H. (1920). *Studies in neurology.* London: Hodder Stoughton.

Head, S., Williamson, D. A., Duchmann, E. G., & Bennett, R. (1988, November). *Bulimia nervosa: Association with axis I and axis II disorders.* Poster presented to the Annual Meeting for the Association for the Advancement of Behavior Therapy, 1988.

Herman, C. P. & Polivy, J. (1975). Anxiety, restraint and eating behavior. *Journal of Abnormal Psychology, 84,* 666–672.

Herman, C. P. & Polivy, J. (1980). Restrained eating. In A. J. Stunkard (Ed.), *Obesity* (pp. 208–225). Philadelphia: W. B. Saunders Co.

Hinz, L. D. & Williamson, D. A. (1987). Bulimia and depression: A review of the affective variant hypothesis. *Psychological Bulletin, 102,* 150–158.

Hirsch, J. & Knittle, J. L. (1970). Cellularity of obese and nonobese human adipose tissue. *Federation Proceedings, 29,* 1516–1521.

Hodgson, R. J. & Rachman, S. (1977). Obsessional-compulsive complaints. *Behaviour Research and Therapy, 15,* 389–395.

Hood, J., Moore, T. E., & Garner, D. M. (1982). Locus of control as a measure of ineffectiveness in anorexia nervosa. *Journal of Consulting and Clincial Psychology, 50,* 3–13.

Hsu, L. K. G., Crisp, A. H., & Harding, B. (1979). Outcome of anorexia nervosa. *Lancet, 1:8107,* 61–65.

Hsu, L. K. G., Meltzer, E. S., & Crisp, A. H. (1981). Schizophrenia and anorexia nervosa. *Journal of Nervous and Mental Disease, 169,* 273–276.

Hudson, J. I., Pope, H. G., Yurgelun-Todd, D., Jonas, J. M., & Frankenburg, F. R. (1987). A controlled study of lifetime prevalence of affective and other psychiatric disorders in bulimic outpatients. *American Journal of Psychiatry, 144,* 1283–1287.

Hudson, J. I., Weiss, R. D., Pope, H. G., McElroy, S. L., & Mirin, S. M. (in press). Eating disorders in hospitalized substance abusers. *Journal of Clinical Psychiatry.*

Johnson, C. & Larson, R. (1982). Bulimia: An analysis of moods and behavior. *Psychosomatic Medicine, 44,* 341–351.

Johnson, C., Lewis, C., Love, S., Lewis, L., & Stuckey, M. (1984). Incidence and correlates of bulimic behavior in a female high school population. *Journal of Youth and Adolescence, 13,* 15–26.

Johnson, C., Stuckey, M. K., Lewis, L. D., & Schwartz, D. M. (1983). Bulimia: A descriptive study of 316 cases. *International Journal of Eating Disorders, 2,* 3–16.

Johnson, P. R. & Hirsch, J. (1972). Cellularity of adipose depots in six strains of genetically obese mice. *Journal of Lipid Research, 13,* 2–11.

Johnson, W. G., Corrigan, S. A., & Mayo, L. L. (1987). Innovative treatment approaches to bulimia nervosa. *Behavior Modification, 11,* 373–388.

Johnson, W. G., & Stalonas, P. M. (1981). *Weight no longer.* Gretna, LA: Pelican Publishing.

Kanner, A. D., Coyne, J. C., Schaefer, C., & Lazarus, R. S. (1981). Comparison of two modes of stress measurement: Daily hassles and uplifts versus major life events. *Journal of Behavioral Medicine, 4,* 1–39.

Kapur, B. M. & Israel, Y. (1983). A dipstick methodology for rapid determination for ethanol and methanol. *Clinical Biochemistry, 17,* 201.

Kasvikis, Y. G., Tsakiris, F., Marks, I. M., Basoglu, M., & Noshirvani, H. F. (1986). Past history of anorexia nervosa in women with obsessive-compulsive disorder. *International Journal of Eating Disorders, 5,* 1069–1075.

Katzman, M. A. & Wolchik, S. A. (1984). Bulimia and binge eating in college women: A comparison of personality and behavioral characteristics. *Journal of Consulting and Clinical Psychology, 52,* 423–428.

Keesey, R. E. (1980). A set-point analysis of the regulation of body weight. In A. J. Stunkard (Ed.), *Obesity* (pp. 144–165). Philadelphia: W. B. Saunders Company.

Kirkley, B., Agras, W. S., & Weiss, J. J. (1985). Nutritional inadequacy in the diets of treated bulimics. *Behavior Therapy, 16,* 287–291.

Krotkiewski, M., Sjostrom, L., Bjorntorp, P., Carlgren, G., Garellick, G., & Smith, U. (1977). Adipose tissue cellularity in relation to prognosis for weight reduction. *International Journal of Obesity, 1,* 395–416.

Lacey, H. G. (1983). Bulimia nervosa, binge eating and psychogenic vomiting: A controlled treatment study and long-term outcome. *British Medical Journal, 286,* 1609–1613.

La Tourette, G. de. (1895). *G.A.E.B.: Traite cliníque et thérapeutic de l'hystéric.* [Clinical traits and therapy of the hysteric]. Paris: Plou, Nouit, et Co.

Lee, N. F., Rush, A. J., & Mitchell, J. E. (1985). Bulimia and depression. *Journal of Affective Disorders, 9,* 231–238.

Leon, G. R., Lucas, A. R., Colligan, R. C., Ferdinande, R. J., & Kamp, J. (1985). Sexual, body-image, and personality attitudes in anorexia nervosa. *Journal of Abnormal Child Psychology, 13,* 245–258.

MacPhillamy, D. J. & Lewinsohn, P. M. (1974). Depression as a function of levels of desired and obtained pleasure. *Journal of Abnormal Psychology, 83,* 651–657.

MacPhillamy, D. J. & Lewinsohn, P. M. (1976). *Manual for the pleasant events schedule.* Unpublished manuscript, University of Oregon.

Marcus, M. D. & Wing, R. R. (1987). Binge eating among the obese. *Annals of Behavioral Medicine, 9,* 23–27.

Marlatt, G. A. (1976). The drinking profile—A questionnaire for the behavioral assesssment of alcoholism. In E. J. Mash & L. G. Terdal (Eds.), *Behavior therapy assessment: Diagnosis, design and evaluation* (pp. 121–137). New York: Springer.

Metropolitan Life Foundation. (1983). 1983 Metropolitan height and weight tables. *Statistical Bulletin, 64,* 2–9.

Miller, D. S. (1975). Overfeeding in man. In G. A. Bray (Ed.), *Obesity in perspective* (pp. 137–143). Washington, DC: U.S. Government Printing Office.

Millon, T. (1982). *Millon Clinical Multiaxial Inventory* (2nd ed.). Minneapolis: National Computer Systems.

Minuchin, S., Rosman, B. L., & Baker, L. (1978). *Psychosomatic families: Anorexia nervosa in context.* Cambridge, MA: Harvard University Press.

Mitchell, J. E., Pyle, R. L., Hatsukami, D., & Eckert, E. D. (1986). What are atypical eating disorders? *Psychosomatics, 27,* 21–28.

Moos, R. H. & Moos, B. S. (1980). *Family environment scale.* Palo Alto: Consulting Psychologists Press.

Moos, R. H. & Moos, B. S. (1986). *Family environment scale* (2nd ed.). Palo Alto: Consulting Psychologists Press.

National Center for Health Statistics: Plan and operation of the HANE Survey, United States 1971–1973. Washington, DC: National Center for Health Statistics, 1973. (Vital and Health Statistics, series 1, no. 10a and 10b.) (DHEW publ no. [HSM] 73-1310.)

Newark, C. S. (1979). *MMPI: Clinical and research trends.* New York: Praeger.

Norris, D. L. (1984). The effects of mirror confrontation on self-estimation of body dimensions in anorexia nervosa, bulimia, and two control groups. *Psychological Medicine, 14,* 835–842.

Norvell, N. & Cooley, E. (1987). Diagnostic issues in eating disorders: Two cases of atypical eating disorder. *International Journal of Psychiatry in Medicine, 16,* 317–323.

Palmer, R., Christie, M., Cordle, C., Davis, D., & Kendrick, J. (1987). The Clinical Eating Disorder Rating Instrument (CEDRI): A preliminary description. *International Journal of Eating Disorders, 6,* 9–16.

Perkins, K. A., McKenzie, S. J., & Stoney, C. M. (1987). The relevance of metabolic rate in behavioral medicine research. *Behavior Modification, 11,* 286–311.

Pierloot, R. A. & Houben, M. E. (1978). Estimation of body dimensions in anorexia nervosa. *Psychological Medicine, 8,* 317–324.

Piersma, H. L. (1986). The factor structure of the Millon Multiaxial Clinical Inventory (MCMI). *Journal of Personality Assessment, 50,* 578–584.

Piran, N., Lerner, P., Garfinkel, P. E., Kennedy, S. H., & Brouillete, C. (1988). Personality disorders in anorexic patients. *International Journal of Eating Disorders, 7,* 589–599.

Polivy, J. & Herman, C. P. (1985). Dieting and binging: A causal analysis. *American Psychologist, 40,* 193–201.

Pope, H. G., & Hudson, J. I. (1985). Biological treatments of eating disorders. In S. W. Emmett (Ed.), *Theory and treatment of anorexia nervosa and bulimia: Biomedical, sociocultural, and psychosocial perspectives.* New York: Brunner/Mazel.

Prather, R. C. (1989). *The affective variant hypothesis: How is bulimia nervosa related to depression?* Unpublished doctoral dissertation, Louisiana State University, Baton Rouge, LA.

Prather, R. C. & Williamson, D. A. (1988). Psychopathology associated with bulimia, binge eating, and obesity. *International Journal of Eating Disorders, 7,* 177–184.

Price, R. A. (1987). Genetics of human obesity. *Annals of Behavioral Medicine, 9,* 9–14.

Pudel, V. E. (1977). Human feeding in the laboratory. In G. A. Bray (Ed.), *Recent advances in obesity research: II* (pp. 66–75). Los Angeles: Newman Publishing.

Pyle, R. L., Mitchell, J. E., & Eckert, E. D. (1981). Bulimia: A report of 34 cases. *Journal of Clinical Psychiatry, 42,* 60–64.

Pyle, R. L., Mitchell, J. E., & Eckert, E. D. (1986). The use of weight tables to categorize patients with eating disorders. *International Journal of Eating Disorders, 5,* 377–383.

Redloff, L. S. (1977). The CES-D scale: A self-report depression scale for research in the general population. *Applied Psychological Measurement, 1,* 385–401.

Reitman, E. E. & Cleveland, S. E. (1964). Changes in body image following sensory deprivation in schizophrenic and control groups. *Journal of Abnormal and Social Psycology, 68,* 168–176.

Rosen, J. C. & Leitenberg, H. (1982). Bulimia nervosa: Treatment with exposure and response prevention. *Behavior Therapy, 13,* 117–124.

Rosen, J. C., Leitenberg, H., Fondacaro, K. M., Gross, J., & Willmuth, M. E. (1985). Standardized test meals in assessment of eating behavior in bulimia nervosa: Consumption of feared foods when vomiting is prevented. *International Journal of Eating Disorders, 4,* 59–70.

Ruderman, A. J. & Wilson, G. T. (1979). Weight, restraint, cognitions, and counterregulation. *Behavior Research and Therapy, 17,* 581–590.

Ruff, G. A. & Barrios, B. A. (1986). Realistic assessment of body image. *Behavioral Assessment, 8,* 237–251.

Ruggiero, L., Williamson, D. A., Davis, C. J., Schlundt, D. G., & Carey, M. P. (1988). Forbidden food survey: Measure of bulimic's anticipated emotional reactions to specific foods. *Addictive Behaviors, 13,* 267–174.

Russell, G. F. M. (1979). Bulimia nervosa: An ominous variety of anorexia nervosa. *Psychological Medicine, 9,* 429–448.

Salaspuro, M. (1986). Conventional and coming laboratory markers of alcoholism and heavy drinking. *Alcoholism: Clinical and Experimental Research, 10,* (supplement), 5S–10S.

Schilder, P. (1935). *Image and appearance of the human body.* London: Kegan, Paul, Trench, Trubner, and Company.

Schlundt, D. G. (1989). Assessment of eating behavior in bulimia nervosa: The self-monitoring analysis system. In W. G. Johnson (Ed.), *Advances in Eating Disorders, Vol II.* (pp. 1–41). New York: JAI Press.

Schlundt, D. G. & Bell, C. (1988, November). *BITS: A microcomputer program for assessing cognitive and affective components of body image.* Paper presented at the annual meeting of the Association for Advancement of Behavior Therapy, New York.

Schlundt, D. G. & Johnson, W. G. (in press). *Assessment and treatment of anorexia and bulimia nervosa.* Needham Heights, MA: Allyn & Bacon.

Schlundt, D. G., Johnson, W. G., & Jarrell, M. P. (1985). A naturalistic functional analysis of eating behavior in bulimia and obesity. *Advances in Behavior Research and Therapy, 7,* 149–162.

Schlundt, D. G., Johnson, W. G., & Jarrell, M. P. (1986). A sequential analysis of environmental, behavioral, and affective variables predictive of vomiting in bulimia nervosa. *Behavioral Assessment, 8,* 253–269.

Schotte, D. E. & Stunkard, A. J. (1987). Bulimia vs. bulimic behaviors on a college campus. *Journal of the American Medical Association, 258,* 1213–1215.

Secord, P. F. & Jourard, S. M. (1953). The appraisal of body-cathexis: Body-cathexis and the self. *Journal of Consulting Psychology, 17,* 343–347.

Seime, R. J., Weiner, A. L., & Fremouw, W. J. (1988, November). *Body image distortion and dissatisfaction in bulimic patients and women at high and low risk for bulimia.* Presented at the annual meeting of the Association for the Advancement of Behavior Therapy, New York.

Selzer, M. L. (1971). Michigan Alcoholism Screening Test. The quest for a new diagnostic instrument. *American Journal of Psychiatry, 127,* 1653–1658.

Sjostrom, L. (1980). Fat cells and body weight. In A. J. Stunkard (Ed.), *Obesity* (pp. 72–100). Philadelphia: W. B. Saunders Company.

Sjostrom, L. & Bjorntorp, P. (1974). Body composition and adipose tissue cellularity in human obesity. *Acta Medica Scandinavia, 195,* 201–211.

Skinner, H. A. (1982). The drug abuse screening test. *Addictive Behaviors, 7,* 363–371.

Slade, P. D. (1977). Awareness of body dimensions during pregnancy: An analogue study. *Psychological Medicine, 7,* 245–252.

Slade, P. D. & Russell, G. F. M. (1973). Awareness of body dimensions in anorexia nervosa: Cross-sectional and longitudinal studies. *Psychological Medicine, 3,* 188–199.

Small, A. C., Madero, J., Gross, H., Teagno, L., Leib, J., & Ebert, M. (1981). *Journal of Clinical Psychology, 37,* 733–736.

Smith, M. C. & Thelen, M. H. (1984). Development and validation of a test for bulimia. *Journal of Consulting and Clinical Psychology, 52,* 863–872.

Snyder, D. K. (1979). Multidimensional assessment of marital satisfaction. *Journal of Marriage and the Family, 41,* 121–131.

Sobell, L. C., Maisto, S. A., Sobell, M. B., & Cooper, A. M. (1979). Reliability of alcohol abusers' self-reports of drinking behavior. *Behaviour Research and Therapy, 17,* 157–160.

Sobell, L. C. & Sobell, M. B. (1986). Can we do without self-reports? *The Behavior Therapist, 9,* 141–146.

Sobell, M. B. & Sobell, L. C. (1975). A brief technical report on the mobat: An inexpensive portable test for determining blood alcohol concentration. *Journal of Applied Behavior Analysis, 8,* 117–120.

Spanier, G. B. (1976). Measuring dyadic adjustment: New scales for assessing the quality of marriage and similar dyads. *Journal of Marriage and the Family, 38,* 15–28.

Speilberger, C. D., Gorsuch, R. L., & Lushene, R. E. (1970). *Manual for the state-trait anxiety inventory.* Palo Alto, CA: Consulting Psychologists Press.

Spitzer, R. L., Endicott, J., & Robins, E. (1975). Research diagnostic criteria. *Psychopharmicologia Bulletin, 11,* 22–25.

Spitzer, R. L., Endicott, J., & Robins, E. (1978). Research diagnostic criteria: Rationale and reliability. *Archives of General Psychiatry, 36,* 773–782.

Stevens, E. V. & Salisbury, J. D. (1984). Group therapy for bulimic adults. *American Journal of Orthopsychiatry, 54,* 156–161.

Stordy, B. J., Marks, V., Kalucy, R. S., & Crisp, A. H. (1977). Weight gain, thermic effects of glucose, and resting metabolic rate during recovery from anorexia nervosa. *American Journal of Clinical Nutrition, 30,* 138–146.

Strober, M., Goldenberg, I., Green, J., & Saxon, J. (1979). Body image disturbance during the acute and recuperative phase. *Psychological Medicine, 9,* 695–701.

Strober, M. & Humphrey, L. L. (1987). Familial contributions to the etiology and course of anorexia nervosa and bulimia. *Journal of Consulting and Clinical Psychology, 55,* 654–659.

Telch, C. F., Agras, W. S., & Rossiter, E. M. (1988). Binge eating increases with increasing adiposity. *International Journal of Eating Disorders, 7,* 115–120.

Theander, S. (1970). Anorexia nervosa: A psychiatric investigation of 94 female patients. *Acta Psychiatrica Scandinavia, 214,* 1–194.

Thelen, M. H., Mann, L. M., Pruitt, J., & Smith, M. (1987). Bulimia: Prevalence and component factors in college women. *Journal of Psychosomatic Research, 31,* 73–78.

Thompson, J. K. & Thompson, C. M. (1986). Body size distortion and self-esteem in asymptomatic, normal weight males and females. *International Journal of Eating Disorders, 5,* 1061–1068.

Touyz, S. W., Beumont, P. J. V., Collins, J. K., & Cowie, I. (1985). Body shape perception in bulimia and anorexia nervosa. *International Journal of Eating Disorders, 4,* 259–265.

Touyz, S. W., Beumont, P. J. V., Collins, J. K., McCabe, M., & Jupp, J. (1984). Body shape perception and its disturbance in anorexia nervosa. *British Journal of Psychiatry, 144,* 167–171.

Traub, A. C. & Orbach, J. (1964). Psychophysical studies of body image: I. The adjustable distorting mirror. *Archives of General Psychiatry, 11,* 53–66.

Van Buren, D. & Williamson, D. A. (1988). Marital relationships and conflict resolution skills of bulimics. *International Journal of Eating Disorders, 7,* 735–741.

Watson, D. & Friend, R. (1969). Measurement of social-evaluative anxiety. *Journal of Consulting and Clinical Psychology, 33,* 371–375.

Webster, J. D., Hesp, R., & Garrow, J. S. (1984). The composition of excess weight in obese women estimated by body density, total body water, and total body potassium. *Human Nutrition: Clinical Nutrition, 38,* 299–306.

Weiss, S. R. & Ebert, M. H. (1983). Psychological and behavioral characteristics of normal-weight bulimics and normal-weight controls. *Psychosomatic Medicine, 45,* 293–303.

Weissman, A. & Beck, A. T. (1978, November). *Development and validation of the Dysfunctional Attitude Scale (DAS).* Paper presented at the 12th annual meeting for the Association for the Advancement of Behavior Therapy, Chicago.

Williamson, D. A., Davis, C. J., Goreczny, A. J., Bennett, S. M., & Gleaves, D. H. (in press). Development of a simple procedure for assessing body image disturbances. *Behavioral Assessment.*

Williamson, D. A., Davis, C. J., Goreczny, A. J., McKenzie, S. J., & Watkins, P. C. (1989). The eating questionnaire-revised: A new symptom checklist for bulimia. In P. A. Keller & L. G. Ritt (Eds.), *Innovations in clinical pratice: A sourcebook* (pp. 321–326). Sarasota, FL: Professional Resource Exchange, Inc.

Williamson, D. A., Davis, C. J., Goreczny, A. J., & Blouin, D. C. (1989). Body image disturbances in bulimia nervosa: Influences of actual body size. *Journal of Abnormal Psychology, 98,* 97–99.

Williamson, D. A., Davis, C. J., & Ruggiero, L. (1987). Eating disorders. In R. L. Morrison & A. S. Bellack (Eds.), *Medical factors and psychological disorders: A handbook for psychologists* (pp. 351–370). New York: Plenum.

Williamson, D. A., Goreczny, A. J., Davis, C. J., Ruggiero, L., & McKenzie, S. J. (1988). Psychophysiological analysis of the anxiety model of bulimia nervosa. *Behavior Therapy, 19,* 1–9.

Williamson, D. A., Kelley, M. L., Cavell, T. A., & Prather, R. C. (1987). Eating and eliminating disorders. In C. L. Frame & J. L. Matson (Eds.), *Handbook of assessment in childhood psychology: Applied issues in differential diagnosis and treatment evaluation* (pp. 461–487). New York: Plenum.

Williamson, D. A., Kelley, M. L., Davis, C. J., Ruggiero, L., & Blouin, D. C. (1985). Psychopathology of eating disorders: A controlled comparison of bulimic, obese, and normal subjects. *Journal of Consulting and Clinical Psychology, 53,* 161–166.

Williamson, D. A., Lawson, O. D., Bennett, S. M., & Hinz, L. (1989). Behavioral treatment of night binging and rumination in an adult case of bulimia nervosa. *Journal of Behavior Therapy and Experimental Psychiatry, 20,* 73–77.

Williamson, D. A., Prather, R. C., Goreczny, A. J., Davis, C. J., & McKenzie, S. J. (1989). A comprehensive model of bulimia nervosa: Empirical evaluation. In W. G. Johnson (Ed.), *Advances in eating disorders* (pp. 137–156). Greenwich, CT: JAI Press.

Williamson, D. A., Prather, R. C., Upton, L., Davis, C. J., Ruggiero, L., & Van Buren, D. (1987). Severity of bulimia: Relationship with depression and other psychopathology. *International Journal of Eating Disorders, 6,* 39–47.

Willmuth, M. E., Leitenberg, H., Rosen, J. C., Fondacaro, K. M., & Gross, J. (1985). Body size distortion in bulimia nervosa. *International Journal of Eating Disorders, 4,* 71–78.

Wilson, G. T. & Lindholm, L. (1987). Bulimia nervosa and depression. *International Journal of Eating Disorders, 6,* 725–732.

Wingate, B. A. & Christie, M. J. (1978). Ego strength and body image in anorexia nervosa. *Journal of Psychosomatic Research, 22,* 201–204.

Winstead, B. A. & Cash, T. F. (1984, March). *Reliability and validity of the Body-Self Relations Questionnaire: A new measure of body image.* Paper presented at the meeting of the Southeastern Psychological Association, New Orleans, LA.

Woody, E. Z., Costanzo, P. R., Leifer, H., & Conger, J. (1981). The effects of taste and caloric perceptions on the eating behavior of restrained and unrestrained subjects. *Cognitive Therapy and Research, 5,* 381–390.

Interview for Diagnosis of Eating Disorders (IDED)

DATE _____
NAME _____ AGE _____ RACE _____
DATE OF BIRTH _____ WEIGHT _____ HEIGHT _____
ADDRESS _____
TELEPHONE _____ REFERRED BY _____

I. *General Assessment and History*

1. What types of problems do you have with eating or weight-related matters? How long has this been a problem?

2. What has been your highest and lowest weight? When?

3. Were you overweight as a child?   Y   N   (Describe.)

4. Were you/are you overweight as an adolescent?   Y   N
   (Describe.)

5. What has been the course of your eating problems? (How the behavior began, increases, decreases, changes in eating.)

6. Have you had any medical/dental problems? (Check for dizziness, LBP, HBP, tooth erosion, thyroid problems, diabetes.)

7. Do you avoid eating certain foods?   Y   N   (Describe.)

   What emotional reaction occurs when you eat these "forbidden" foods? (Foods which are avoided or purged due to a belief that the foods will lead to rapid and significant weight gain.)

8. How many members are there in your household?

   Do they know about your eating problems?   Y   N
   If yes, how do they react/feel about your eating disorder?

Would they participate in your treatment?

II. *Anorexia Nervosa*

1. Do you currently go periods of time without eating (starvation) to control your weight?   Y   N   (If Y, describe.)

   When did you first begin to lose weight/restrict your eating?

   Are there any factors/situations which seem to increase or decrease periods of restrictive eating?

2. Do you feel that your weight is normal?   Y   N   (Describe.)

3. What emotional reaction would you have if you lost
   2 lbs.?

   5 lbs.?

   10 lbs.?

   What emotional reaction would you have if you gained
   2 lbs.?

   5 lbs.?

   10 lbs.?

4. Do you wish to be thinner than you are now?   Y   N
(If Y, ask what body areas should be thinner.)

What is your goal weight?

Do you think or worry a lot about your weight and body size?

Do you often feel "fat" when you gain only a few pounds?   Y   N
(Describe.)

Do you weigh yourself often?   Y   N   How often?

5. When was your last menstrual cycle?

Have you experienced menstrual irregularities within the last three
months?   Y   N   (Describe.)

III. *Bulimia Nervosa*

1. Do you ever binge (rapid consumption of large amounts of food in a
discrete period of time)? What is the daily course of your binge eating?
(Describe all covert and overt events that usually occur prior to, during, and after a binge.)

Do you ever feel as though you have overeaten when you eat small
portions of certain fattening foods?   Y   N   (Describe.)

When did you first begin to have problems with binging?

Are there any factors which appear to increase or decrease the frequency of binge eating?

2. Do you feel out of control prior to or during a binge?   Y   N
   (Describe.) Do you feel hungry prior to a binge?   Y   N

3. Do you purge after meals or after a binge?   Y   N

   Do you vomit?   Y   N   How often per day/week?

   Do you use laxatives?   Y   N   How often, what type?

   Do you use diuretics?   Y   N   How often, what type?

   Do you use appetite suppressants?   Y   N   How often, what type?

   Do you often go on strict diets?   Y   N   How often, what type?

   Do you engage in vigorous exercise?   Y   N   How often, what type?

   When did you first begin to purge?

   Are there any factors which appear to increase or decrease the frequency of purging?

4. How often does the binge eating occur?

How long have you been binging at least twice per week?

How often does the binge-purge cycle occur?

IV. *Compulsive Overeating*

1. If you binge, what types of food do you typically eat?

2. Do you binge alone, or in secret?   Y   N   (Describe.)

3. What emotions typically precede a binge?

4. Do you often attempt to diet in order to lose weight? (Describe.)

5. Have you had frequent weight fluctuations greater than 10 pounds in the past few years?   Y   N   (Describe.)

6. Do you consider your eating to be abnormal?   Y   N
   Do you feel that you have control over your eating?   Y   N

7. How do you feel during and after a binge episode? (Describe.)

8. Are you satisfied with your current weight?   Y   N

   If no, what is your weight goal?

Appendix B
Rating Scale for the IDED

I. *Anorexia Nervosa*

1. Refusal to maintain appropriate weight for height

1	2	3	4	5	6	7
Accepts normal weight	Prefers 5% below normal weight	Prefers 10% below normal weight	Prefers 15% below normal weight	Prefers 20% below normal weight	Prefers 25% below normal weight	Prefers greater than 25% below normal weight

2. Intense fear of weight gain

1	2	3	4	5	6	7
No Problem	Minimal Problem	Minimal Fear	Moder-ate Fear	Strong Fear	Intense Fear	Morbid Fear

3. Body image disturbance: Feels "fat" even though not significantly overweight

1	2	3	4	5	6	7
Never	Occa-sion-ally when "stuffed"	After eating meals	After eating small amounts of food	Most of the time	Almost all of time	All of the time

172

4. Amenorrhea

1	2	3	4	5	6	7
Very Regular	Slight Irregu- larity	Missed 2 cycles last 6 months	Missed 3 cycles last 6 months	Missed 4 cycles last 6 months	Missed 5 cycles last 6 months	Missed 6 cycles last 6 months

II. *Bulimia Nervosa*

1. Recurrent binge-eating episodes

1	2	3	4	5	6	7
Never binges	Infre- quent and small	Infre- quent but large	Frequent and large	Frequent includ- ing binges and for- bidden foods	Very fre- quent w/ only large binges	Very fre- quent w/ binges plus for- bidden foods

2. Feeling of loss of control during binge eating

1	2	3	4	5	6	7
Always in control	Rare loss of control	Occa- sional loss of control	Frequent loss of control	Usually out of control	Almost always out of control	Never in control

3. Purgative behavior

1	2	3	4	5	6	7
None	Purges 1–2 times/ year	Purges 1 time/3 months	Purges 1–3 times/ month	Purges 1–2 times/ week	Purges 3–6 times/ week	Purges 1 or more times/ day

4. Frequency of binge eating

1	2	3	4	5	6	7
Rarely occurs	Occurs a few times/ year	1–4 times/ month	5–8 times/ month	2–3 times/ week	4–6 times/ week	Occurs daily or almost daily

5. Overconcern with body shape and size

1	2	3	4	5	6	7
No over-concern	Minimal concern	Some preoc-cupation	Mode-rate degree of preoc-cupation	Preoc-cupied most of the time	Preoc-cupied almost all of the time	Preoc-cupied all of the time

III. *Compulsive Overeating*

1. Frequency of recurrent binge-eating episodes

1	2	3	4	5	6	7
Never Binges	Binges less than once per month	Binges once per week or less	Binges about twice per week	Binges 3 to 6 times per week	Binges once per day	Usually binges more than once per day

2. Consumption of high-calorie, easily ingested food during a binge

1	2	3	4	5	6	7
No binges	Minimal Overeat of nor-mal foods	Moder-ate Overeat of nor-mal foods	Binges on nor-mal foods	Binges on nor-mal and hi-cal foods	Binges exclu-sively on hi-cal foods	Overeats at meals and binges only on hi-cal foods

3. Inconspicuous eating during a binge

1	2	3	4	5	6	7
No binges	Prefers to eat with friends or family	Overeats with friends or family	Binges with few people	Binges at home alone with others in house	Rarely binges with anyone else present	Binges only when alone

4. Repeated efforts at dieting

1	2	3	4	5	6	7
Never diets	Diets 1–2 times/ year	Diets 3–4 times/ year	Diets 5–6 times/ year	Diets every month	Diets almost every week	Diets all of the time

5. Negative affect prior to binge

1	2	3	4	5	6	7
No binges	Seldom overeats due to negative affect	Sometimes overeats due to negative affect	Often binges due to negative affect	Usually binges due to negative affect	Almost always binges due to negative affect	Always binges due to negative affect

6. Frequent weight fluctuations greater than 10 lbs.

1	2	3	4	5	6	7
None	Minimal weight fluctuation	Few 1–9 lbs.	Few 10 lbs.	Many 10 lbs.	Few 10–20 lbs.	Many 10–20 lbs.

7. Absence of purgative behaviors

._____._____._____._____._____._____._____

1	2	3	4	5	6	7
Purges daily	Purges weekly	Purges monthly	Purges Infrequently	Purges 1–2 times/ year	Diets occasionally	None

8. Realization that eating pattern is abnormal/out of control

._____._____._____._____._____._____._____

1	2	3	4	5	6	7
No problem	Minimal problem	Occasional mild feelings	Frequent mild feelings	Frequent moderate feelings	Frequent intense feelings	Extremely frequent and intense

9. Depressed mood and self-deprecating thoughts after a binge

._____._____._____._____._____._____._____

1	2	3	4	5	6	7
No binges	No depression post-binge	Minimal depression post-binge	Modest depression post-binge	Moderate depression post-binge	Severe depression post-binge	Extreme depression post-binge

10. Body size dissatisfaction

._____._____._____._____._____._____._____

1	2	3	4	5	6	7
Never	Occasional when "stuffed"	After eating meals	After eating small amounts of food	Most of the time	Almost all of the time	All of the time

Appendix C
Brief Interview of Secondary Psychopathology (BISP)

DEPRESSION AND ANXIETY

The following questions relate to the areas of both anxiety and depression. Pages 180–184 list the various symptom categories relating to both anxiety and depression and are grouped by disorder. The letters and numbers preceding each question group correspond with the rating scales found on pages 180–184. For example D:1 refers to Depression rating scale 1 and A:1 refers to Anxiety rating scale 1. Following the interview a total score for anxiety and depression severity may be recorded by totaling the clinician ratings for the appropriate symptom groups. If the patient receives a total score of greater than 6 for anxiety the interviewer should investigate further for specific anxiety disorders. If the patient achieves a score of greater than 10 on depression, it is recommended that a diagnosis of dysthymia be further evaluated; if the clinician's ratings total 16 or greater on depression items, a diagnosis of major depression should be ruled out via further diagnostic evaluation.

All ratings should be made for the past month. The interviewer should make this known to the patient, and may wish to reference this time period with notable dates. For example, a clinician conducting an interview on January 10 may wish to say:

All of the following questions are for the past month only. That would be from December 10 until today. That means that Christmas, New Year's, and I believe your anniversary were celebrated in this time period we will be discussing.

MOOD D:1, 2, A:12, 13. How have you been feeling lately? What has your mood been like? Have you been worried or upset? Have you felt any anxiety or panic (describe symptoms)?

If patient reports anxiety symptoms, ask the following question: Does the anxiety occur at any particular time, place or situation? Are there any situatons you avoid because they make you nervous or scared?

SLEEP D:3, A:14. Do you have trouble falling asleep? Do you wake often during the night? Do you wake early in the morning before you would like to? Can you get back to sleep? Are you sleeping more than usual? How much? Do you usually take naps during the day? For how long?

SOMATIC/APPETITE D:4, A:15, 16. Have you noticed any changes in your body lately? Have you been constipated? Have you noticed changes in your heart rate or breathing? How has your appetite been? Have you had trouble eating? Is this related to your mood?

OBSESSIVE-COMPULSIVE A:17. Have you had trouble with your thoughts? Do you ever have thoughts that bother you but you can't seem to get rid of them? Do you ever seem compelled to do something? Do you have any ritualistic habits (give examples)?

ACTIVITY/INTEREST D:5, 6, 7. Has it been hard to go out and do things lately? Do you have to push yourself? Do you seem to tire easily? Are you as interested in things as you used to be? Do you get as much pleasure out of things as you used to? Is there anything that you still enjoy?

HOPELESSNESS D:8. Do you think that things will get better? What does the future look like? Does anything lift your spirits or encourage you anymore?

WORTHLESSNESS D:9. How do you feel about yourself? Do you have a tendency to get down on yourself? What is your self-esteem like? Do you like yourself? Do you ever feel like a failure? How much of the time?

CONCENTRATION D:10. Have you had trouble concentrating lately? Have you been forgetting things? Have you had trouble making decisions recently?

SUICIDE D:11. Do you feel like life is worth living right now? Have you thought much about death? Have you considered taking your life?

RELATIONSHIPS

Do you like to do things with friends? How often? How many close friends would you say that you have? Are you experiencing any problems with your friends?

Are you married? Are you dating someone regularly? Is this area of your life going well? Would you like it to improve? Are you experiencing any other problems with relatives?

SUBSTANCE USE

Do you like to drink alcohol? How much do you usually drink? How often?

Do you take any prescription or nonprescription drugs? What type? How often?

Has your use of alcohol or drugs ever gotten you into any trouble? Have you ever experienced a blackout? Have you ever received a DWI or DUI? Have you ever received treatment for drug or alcohol related problems?

SYMPTOMS OF DEPRESSION

Circle appropriate rating:

1. Depressed mood

0	1	2	3
not down	reports depression following inquiry	reports feeling sad, down, blue or depressed	depressed mood constant, interferes with activities

2. Anxious mood

0	1	2	3
not worried or anxious	reports some tension following inquiry	reports moderate level of worries, tension, nervousness	anxiety interferes with activities

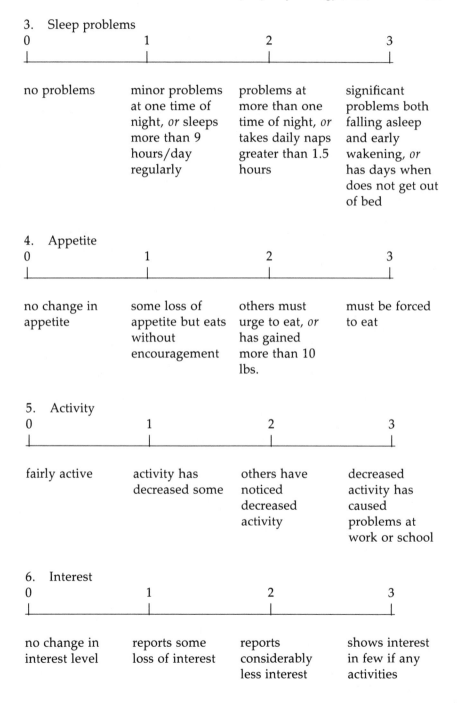

3. Sleep problems

0	1	2	3
no problems	minor problems at one time of night, *or* sleeps more than 9 hours/day regularly	problems at more than one time of night, *or* takes daily naps greater than 1.5 hours	significant problems both falling asleep and early wakening, *or* has days when does not get out of bed

4. Appetite

0	1	2	3
no change in appetite	some loss of appetite but eats without encouragement	others must urge to eat, *or* has gained more than 10 lbs.	must be forced to eat

5. Activity

0	1	2	3
fairly active	activity has decreased some	others have noticed decreased activity	decreased activity has caused problems at work or school

6. Interest

0	1	2	3
no change in interest level	reports some loss of interest	reports considerably less interest	shows interest in few if any activities

7. Anhedonia

0	1	2	3
still enjoys activities	reports some subjective loss of pleasure	reports loss of pleasure in most activities	derives pleasure from few, if any, activities

8. Hopelessness

0	1	2	3
convinced things will improve	things will get better, but not really sure	thinks the future will probably not improve	cannot be encouraged

9. Worthlessness

0	1	2	3
feels as good as most	feels like most are better than they are	volunteers feelings of worthlessness: "no good," "failure," "inferior," "loser"	feelings of worthlessness are fairly pervasive

10. Concentration/indecisiveness

0	1	2	3
no difficulties with decisions or concentration	minor forgetfulness or concentration problems	has problems making decisions	indecisiveness or lack of concentration has resulted in problems at home, work, or school

11. Suicide

0	1	2	3
feels like life is worth living	feels like life is not worth living	has spent time thinking about a suicide plan	any definite suicide attempt

TOTAL DEPRESSION SYMPTOMS: _____

Total greater than 10 = Consider a diagnosis of dysthymia
Total greater than 16 = Consider a diagnosis of major depression

SYMPTOMS OF ANXIETY

12. Anxious mood

0	1	2	3
not worried or anxious	reports some tension following inquiry	reports moderate level of worries, tension, and/or nervousness	anxiety interferes with daily activities

13. Panic

0	1	2	3
no panic symptoms	experiences a few panic symptoms	reports panic attack	has one or more panic attacks per week

14. Sleep problems

0	1	2	3
no difficulty sleeping	minor problems at one time of night	problems at more than one time of night or significant problems at any one time of night	significant problems both falling asleep and early awakening

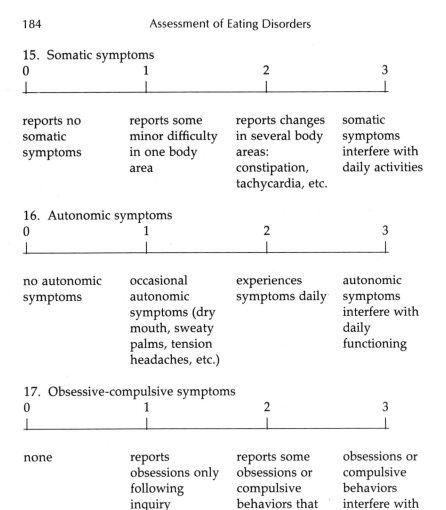

15. Somatic symptoms

0	1	2	3
reports no somatic symptoms	reports some minor difficulty in one body area	reports changes in several body areas: constipation, tachycardia, etc.	somatic symptoms interfere with daily activities

16. Autonomic symptoms

0	1	2	3
no autonomic symptoms	occasional autonomic symptoms (dry mouth, sweaty palms, tension headaches, etc.)	experiences symptoms daily	autonomic symptoms interfere with daily functioning

17. Obsessive-compulsive symptoms

0	1	2	3
none	reports obsessions only following inquiry	reports some obsessions or compulsive behaviors that do not interfere with daily activities	obsessions or compulsive behaviors interfere with daily activities

TOTAL ANXIETY SYMPTOMS ____

Total greater than 6 = Evaluate the presence of an anxiety disorder

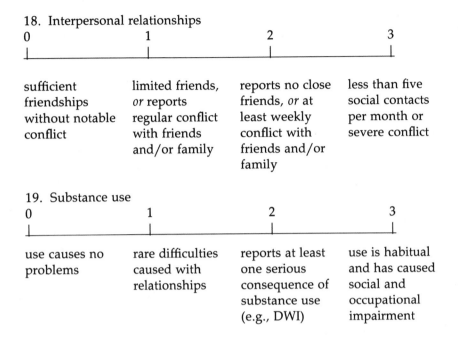

18. Interpersonal relationships

0	1	2	3
sufficient friendships without notable conflict	limited friends, *or* reports regular conflict with friends and/or family	reports no close friends, *or* at least weekly conflict with friends and/or family	less than five social contacts per month or severe conflict

19. Substance use

0	1	2	3
use causes no problems	rare difficulties caused with relationships	reports at least one serious consequence of substance use (e.g., DWI)	use is habitual and has caused social and occupational impairment

Author Index

Subject Index

About the Authors

Donald A. Williamson, Ph.D. is Professor of Psychology and Director of the Psychological Services Center at Louisiana State University. He received his doctorate in clinical psychology in 1978 from Memphis State University and completed a clinical internship at Western Psychiatric Institute and Clinic at the University of Pittsburgh. He has published extensively in the areas of behavior therapy, behavioral medicine, and eating disorders.

C. J. Davis, M.S., M.A. is assistant director of the eating disorders program at Parkland Hospital, Baton Rouge, LA. She is a doctoral candidate in clinical psychology and has completed a clinical internship at Long Beach VA Hospital. Her area of research specialization has concerned behavioral medicine and eating disorders.

Erich G. Duchmann, M.A. is completing a clinical psychology internship at Western Psychiatric Institute and Clinic at the University of Pittsburgh. He is a doctoral candidate in clinical psychology at Louisiana State University. He has research interests in eating disorders and anxiety disorders.

Sandra J. McKenzie, M.A. is a clinical psychology intern at Western Psychiatric Institute and Clinic at the University of Pittsburgh. She is a doctoral candidate in clinical psychology at Louisiana State University. Her research interests are in behavioral medicine and eating disorders.

Philip C. Watkins, M.A. is a doctoral candidate in clinical psychology at Louisiana State University. He is currently on internship at the University of Southern California. His research interests are in depression and eating disorders.

Psychology Practitioner Guidebooks

Editors
Arnold P. Goldstein, Syracuse University
Leonard Krasner, Stanford University & SUNY at Stony Brook
Sol L. Garfield, Washington University in St. Louis

Elsie M. Pinkston & Nathan L. Linsk—CARE OF THE ELDERLY:
A Family Approach

Donald Meichenbaum—STRESS INOCULATION TRAINING

Sebastiano Santostefano—COGNITIVE CONTROL THERAPY WITH
CHILDREN AND ADOLESCENTS

Lillie Weiss, Melanie Katzman & Sharlene Wolchik—TREATING BULIMIA:
A Psychoeducational Approach

Edward B. Blanchard & Frank Andrasik—MANAGEMENT OF CHRONIC
HEADACHES: A Psychological Approach

Raymond G. Romanczyk—CLINICAL UTILIZATION OF
MICROCOMPUTER TECHNOLOGY

Philip H. Bornstein & Marcy T. Bornstein—MARITAL THERAPY:
A Behavioral-Communications Approach

Michael T. Nietzel & Ronald C. Dillehay—PSYCHOLOGICAL
CONSULTATION IN THE COURTROOM

Elizabeth B. Yost, Larry E. Beutler, M. Anne Corbishley & James R.
Allender—GROUP COGNITIVE THERAPY: A Treatment Approach for
Depressed Older Adults

Lillie Weiss—DREAM ANALYSIS IN PSYCHOTHERAPY

Edward A. Kirby & Liam K. Grimley—UNDERSTANDING AND TREATING
ATTENTION DEFICIT DISORDER

Jon Eisenson—LANGUAGE AND SPEECH DISORDERS IN CHILDREN

Eva L. Feindler & Randolph B. Ecton—ADOLESCENT ANGER CONTROL:
Cognitive-Behavioral Techniques

Michael C. Roberts—PEDIATRIC PSYCHOLOGY: Psychological
Interventions and Strategies for Pediatric Problems

Daniel S. Kirschenbaum, William G. Johnson & Peter M. Stalonas, Jr.—
TREATING CHILDHOOD AND ADOLESCENT OBESITY

W. Stewart Agras—EATING DISORDERS: Management of Obesity, Bulimia
and Anorexia Nervosa

Ian H. Gotlib & Catherine A. Colby—TREATMENT OF DEPRESSION:
An Interpersonal Systems Approach

Walter B. Pryzwansky & Robert N. Wendt—PSYCHOLOGY AS A
PROFESSION: Foundations of Practice

Cynthia D. Belar, William W. Deardorff & Karen E. Kelly—THE PRACTICE
OF CLINICAL HEALTH PSYCHOLOGY

Paul Karoly & Mark P. Jensen—MULTIMETHOD ASSESSMENT OF
CHRONIC PAIN